Train y Holistic Hypnotherapy

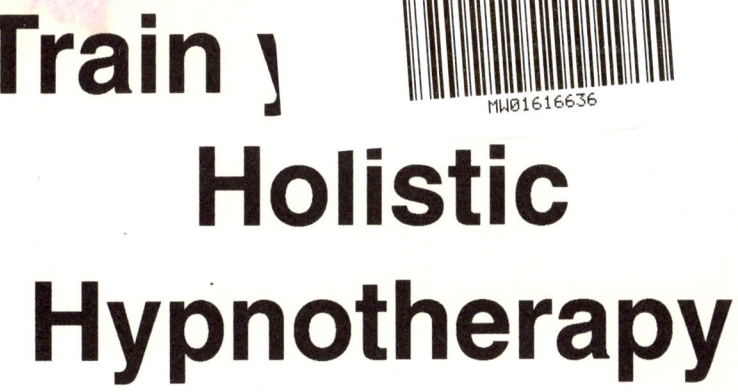

MW01616636

A personal view

by

John Howard

Book Two in a series of Three

(This book should be read in conjunction with the
other two in the series)

First published in Great Britain in 1994

BROOKLYN PUBLISHING GROUP
Moulton Park Business Centre
Northampton NN3 1AQ

Printed and bound in Great Britain by Alden Press Ltd, Oxford.

ISBN 1 898396 05 1
ISBN 1 898396 07 8

British Library Cataloguing-in-Publication Data.
A catalogue record for this book is available from the British Library.

The Author

John Howard has been a highly successful practitioner of hypnotherapy for many years and during this period of time he has healed thousands of people. For several years he lectured on hypnotherapy and the mind in hospitals. He has been retained by one of Britain's largest companies to treat their employees. He has also lectured in colleges, featured in the press, made appearances on 'live' radio and is much in demand as a guest speaker. During personal appearances, he often demonstrates his technique for instant healing.

John is passionately enthusiastic about spreading his knowledge and techniques, by explaining the simple natural healing method that is within everyone. It is this background that lies behind the writing of the three books in the series on training yourself in Holistic Hypnotherapy and the founding of the College of Holistic Hypnotherapy.

Acknowledgments

To my wife and family to whom I owe all. To my friends, colleagues and clients, too numerous to mention and without whose help this series of three hypnotherapy books would not have been written.

Contents

Book Two

Introduction

In my introduction to Book One of this series of books, the concept, that 'something is clearly wrong and something must be missing from today's conventional medicine', was put forward and followed by "But what?" A similar statement and question could be posed and asked about today's society. In theory, we should be living in a more contented world than ever before because we are more knowledgeable than ever; live longer; have more leisure time; and there is no world shortage of food. Yet what are we finding? There is a widespread international and national disharmony, the media in general appear to reveal an unending list of new horrors, and standards seem to be declining in every direction.

We frequently hear of people in senior positions of responsibility, committing all manor of self-discrediting acts; youngsters steal cars, killing and maiming as they *joy-ride*, and wantonly injure or murder innocent and helpless old people. Reports of rapes, sexual assaults and unprovoked attacks are now common place. Police, the seemingly last bastion of public defence, are regularly assaulted and even murdered while carrying out their duties. Indeed, for the first time in Britain some police, and in increasing numbers, are being routinely armed.

We live in a society where many now fear to walk streets, especially after dark. Bank, post office and building society robberies seem commonplace. Theft, mugging and wanton vandalism occur everywhere. Incredible acts of cruelty, injury and awfulness are now carried out by people who frequently seem quite indifferent of the consequences of their acts. On the roads incredible acts of impatience, anger and violence have become common and lead to intimidation, injury and death. In some districts, doctors are reluctant to make home visits, fearful of assaults which have in any case, become almost common in their surgeries. Again, people can now become more spontaneously brutal, angry and lose self-control, far more easily and readily than a few years ago.

This morbid list could be extended almost indefinitely, but it is not necessary to do so, because surely most people are aware that general standards in human relationships are 'mysteriously' declining, and not only in Britain of course, but in most other counties also. People in authority are frequently denying that any fundamental change in society has occurred. They often present statictics to 'prove' their point or to compare modern society with some former times and ages. Perhaps it is just as well that they give us hope and encouragement - after all, if they were to throw their hands in the air and proclaim their dispair and despondency, what then would be the morale of the public? Yet, the man in the street does know, using nothing more complex than his common serse and observation, that something negative is happening to the quality of life and human relatonships, in some general sort of way. Some people blame television, widely available pornographical material, the lack of discipline, unemployment, stress, alcohol, drugs and many other reasons for this decline in society.

Whatever the real cause, something is clearly wrong - but what? The most likely answer is so simple, and surely the people in authority must be aware of it also, but they remain genuinely unable to act. Human judgement, particularly when emotion is involved, has become in some way, impaired and, if so, how or by what?

The amazingly simple answer is most likely to be air pollution. Increasingly, I find people ever more ready to accept this concept; many having arrived at this conclusion for themselves. But if it is this factor whixh is at the heart of the problem. in what way

ii

does it contribute to the result that is occurring? Perhaps the most important ingredient in air pollution is petroleum products particularly where they are directly combusted - millions of tonnes of such products are combusted world-wide and every day. They're burned-off in generators and in industry; exhaust drops on us from aircraft; emitted from countless tonnes of heavy machinery, lorries and cars. Such pollutants are only temporarily visible, mostly at the point of emission but that does not mean they have 'magically' gone away or become ineffectual.

Surely two things must be factual: (a) We must, each and everyone of us, breathe in at least some of this pollution with every breath we draw; and (b) Polluted air must have some effect on us, even if relatively little. The physiological purpose of breathing is to put oxygen into our blood streams, but if that oxygen is contaminated, then that contamination (just as in smoking) will also be circulated within us and eventually some will reach the brain. Whether it could be accumulated there, is for the more scientifically-minded to answer but the fact that it does arrive in the brain cannot be doubted, nor can it be absolutely ruled out that it could have an effect.

The brain itself can be readily effected by even tiny quantities of some chemicals so what then, if every breath draws into the brain such pollution? The most vulnerable part of the mind, to the effects of such pollution, is that part which normally governs and overrides the animalistic subconscious to which there is little concern with right or wrong, moral or immoral considerations. In short, the ability and judgements of the conscious mind could be reduced by such pollution, rather like a single alcoholic drink. In fact a comparison might be made that we are indeed 'intoxicated' by pollution, but unlike alcohol, we are unaware of it.

Pollution pollutes and where it is regularly drawn into the body, who can say it can have no effect on the mind? There is every reason to believe that, if a scientific study were to be made as a means of collating both the growth in the combustion of petroleum products and the apparent deterioration of society, an identifiable link would be found. Lead for example, is known to be highly toxic yet millions of tonnes are regularly pumped into the air through the same combustion process!

Since the beginning of the industrial revolution, pollution has been widespread, especially in Europe. However, human relationships continued to be explainable, given the various conditions of the times, whereas over the past twenty years or so, something inexplicable has occurred. If it is petroleum combustion that is the principle cause of this social decline, then only one long-term prospect for change seems apparent.

This change, perhaps decades away, is for the replacement of our energy needs by electricity but with the product generated through a clean, safe and sustainable nuclear fusion. However, rather than using a nuclear fusion, why not use a current method? Efficient durable batteries, of an acceptable weight, still need to be invented to complete my proposed switch. The technology is suitably advanced for fuelling vehicles and for aircraft to run on combusting hydrogen and oxygen thus producing mainly water as the exhausted output.

Perhaps in this idea lies an easier and quicker solution, albeit costs stand in the way, for currently on price alone for energy basis, petroleum remains unrivalled. While the hypnotherapist can do little in all of this, it is nevertheless useful in helping with a greater understanding of not only what is happening, but also a very possible why? If this mind-distorting pollution factor is being borne by the public at large, it makes the release, if the additional disruptive effects of repression, even more urgent and desirable because surely the pollution effect, coming on top of any repression, could combine to have incalculable consequences?

A Reminiscence

In the autumn of 1946, when I was an eight-year-old, we moved into a modern home. For the first time we actually had a real bathroom - no more tin baths by the fire; trips to an outside toilet or chamber pots under the bed. All-in-all a welcome and marvellous change. On visiting the bathroom from time-to-time during the night I was alarmed and saddened on occasions to see blood-stained 'bandages' in the washbasin left there to soak. Somehow, but I don't know why, I connected them with my mother who was clearly very ill and her illness was making her bleed a lot. I never mentioned my enormous concern to her and she seemed brave enough to pretend to be well. Despite her clever acting though I saw through it and became increasingly afraid. It was only many years later, as I continued to ponder over the mystery, that I realised what I had been witnessing.

In the years immediately following the Second World War, everything was scarce and most things were rationed. Added to this, my stepfather to be held only a poorly paid job on the railways. What my mother had been doing in the bathroom all those years ago was just one of the things with which she had to do to cope. However, with the experiences being repeated they instilled in me a dream that I would grow up and one day discover some great universal healing remedy.

At first I had no idea what that remedy would be, but it would be something that made everyone well no matter what was wrong with them. Since the only treatment I had been given for illness came from a medicine bottle it was obvious to me that my remedy had to be a bottled potion too, but a magical one. I knew nothing of science or medicine and I couldn't wait to grow up for the 'emergency' already existed. Something had to be done now! I realised my only recourse was to begin experimenting immediately; there was no time to be lost. Everything had to be tried, no avenue of exploration could be ignored. I was spurred on in my enthusiasm by the unknown mother who, by using similar research methods, had discovered the bottle her husband used, to oil the small caster wheels on his furniture, was also 'extremely good for small boys. Whilst I always regretted that she had passed her discovery on to my mother, I secretly much admired her initiative.

Somehow I knew that my great remedy would just have to be coloured purple, therefore an added complication clouded the issue. Everything that produced this essential colour was added to my potions. Blackberries were crushed into salt and vinegar with sugar added, just to balance the flavour; blue and pink bath salts were added to milk; bluebell flowers were pulped into rose hip syrup. Some of the neighbours' lilac was stolen but later confiscated by my mother who, on seeing me enter the house with it, proclaimed it unlucky. In fact, it proved only unlucky for me for, in my belief, a vital opportunity and holding much promise, was being denied me. Despite all the setbacks and repeated failures of experiment after experiment I continued with my endeavours.

Then, one day the experimenting was brought to an abrupt halt. Earlier I had heard about just such a fantastic magical ingredient, one I had so far searched for in vain. A friend told me his mother possessed a packet of crystals which turned everything purple. He said that he could steal them and would exchange them for my marbles. The deal was struck with mutual enthusiasm and the contract was eventually fulfilled. I was overjoyed, beyond my wildest hopes, to find that these crystals and just as I had been told they would readily mixed with ordinary tap water to produce copious quantities of stunningly beautiful purple liquid. Surely, I was now hot on the trail; only the finishing touches to my endeavours needed to fall into place. Unfortunately, some of my precious crystals were lost in one experiment when I tried mixing them with glycerine, only to discover that the mixture spontaneously burst into purple flames. The fact that when mixed with water the liquid turned my hands brown, was dismissed by me as only a trifling side effect and one to be ignored. To my unimaginative parents however, the fact that the crystals also turned the washbasin brown, was definitely not to be considered trifling, or to be ignored. An impromptu and heavily biased family court of enquiry was instantly convened. The upshot of which was that I suffered the rough justice of having to reveal the entire contents of my bedroom cupboard laboratory. There would be no appeal against confiscation and no mitigating circumstances were taken into consideration.

It was now the turn of my mother to be alarmed by the array of test tubes, bottles, pillboxes, tins and jars that came to light, one after the other. Great alarm was to be unjustifiably expressed by both parents with the discovery that among my collection of ingredients yet to be experimented with was a small jar of deadly nightshade berries. Looking back and since I had been the only willing guinea pig readily available it is a wonder that I hadn't fatally poisoned myself. Fortunately, the only health cost to me was to feel slightly ill from time to time and occasionally be violently sick.

With my entire laboratory lost, and me now subject to oppressive security checks with my pocket money stopped and the purchasing power of my marbles gone, I had only the laboratory of my mind left. Night after night nothing more dominated my thoughts than that elusive magical elixir. Even in my dreams I sought to solve the problem. Sometimes I did, only annoyingly to awaken, having already forgotten the formula. Eventually both dreams and hopes were to fade and somehow my mother miraculously survived.

Reluctantly, I realised that the search had to be abandoned

and the project, with all its investments, had to be written off. Fortunately the transition was eased by a compensating enthusiasm that was developing in my friend Charlie Price and me to make our very own aircraft from orange boxes. However, my earlier dream was never to leave me entirely. One day in 1985, nearly forty years later, I finally discovered a real elixir. It wasn't purple or even a liquid, instead it came in the form of black letters on white paper. In short, it was a correspondence course on hypnotherapy. This new found 'elixir' couldn't cure everything and everyone but I quickly discovered it did have enormous potential which quickly became realised as I went on course after training course and put the knowledge and instructions that I gained into practice. My forty-year-old dream had finally become all but realised. Since that time, thousands of people have benefited from that knowledge and the enthusiasm for healing that was born in me in those far off earlier days.

It is with enormous joy and satisfaction that, in the pages that have gone and those yet to come, I have attempted to hand over to the reader all that I have come to know of the subject. Realising that in doing so, countless others will benefit from the experience of seemingly 'magical' healing.

FOOTNOTE: Should the reader wish to take up where my own experimentation was abruptly halted, the magical crystals that seemed so near to bringing success, are still readily available today and cost little. Just ask your chemist for a small tub of potassium permanganate. However, he will expect money for them, not marbles. The compensating benefit for this financial requirement is that the crystals can be assumed not to have been stolen so that you will not be faced with the embarrassing prospect of being frog-marched to Aylesbury Street to confront David's angry mother. I have also since discovered they can do wonders in healing foot conditions, albeit in doing so, turn both bowl and feet brown too!

Chapter One

Reincarnation and the Human Spirit

Second only to the difficulty of setting out the chapter on the complexes, this is the most challenging one to write in so much as reincarnation too can be a most highly contested and emotive subject. I never ask anyone to accept what I put forward on this issue, rather taking the position that it is merely presented as a viewpoint or an idea worthy of consideration. More especially, if you should conduct analysis the subject can, and will stray into your work and often quite unexpectedly. If you take the position of refuting reincarnation as a possibility, you will not only have considerably restricted your flexibility, but may have discarded the vital tool that could otherwise have resolved a case. The reincarnation theory suffers the same problem of lacking evidence and provability, as do so many other aspects of dealing with the mind.

However, the lack of hard proof is no guarantee that the theory is disproved or without foundation. On many occasions when all else has failed, it is this theory and how to use it, which has unlocked many cases for me. Before putting the case forward to a client, I ask for their opinion of the possibility of reincarnation and in response most clients report either an existing acceptance of the principle or state they are neutral, holding neither one view nor the other. With tact, it is normally possible to get a client to at least agree to listen to the theory by way of adding to their knowledge and to contribute to their thinking and opinions. Where a stronger rejection of the theory emerges I drop the subject. In any case, the theory is only introduced when some practical objective exists for explaining it. In fact, the subject is raised in about ten percent of cases either by myself or by clients acting on their own initiative. Having the client's interest in hearing it, I begin along the following lines.

The human spirit seems somehow different and separate from the physical body yet part of it, similar in vein to a car and its driver. The car is of little use in the absence of a driver while the driver, without his car, lacks a great deal of certain abilities. When a car eventually 'gives out' through age, wear-and-tear or due to an accident it is not dumped or discarded with the the driver still in it, what usually happens is that the driver obtains a replacement vehicle. So too, when a car is parked at the end of the day, the driver doesn't just sit in it, waiting for the next morning to arrive. Instead he gets out and exists elsewhere. The driver can relax, free of the day's events and gradually becomes tired and the time to sleep arrives. He will sleep until a new day dawns, when once again his routine will recommence.

In many respects, similarities between the body and spirit, and the car and driver, can serve to illustrate the human being. Compared to the garaged car and the driver who leaves it, so too will the spirit tend to leave the 'garaged' or sleeping body. On occasions the body or body's mind may be, or become aware of the spirit departing. For instance, following a hard day, the body may go into sleep quickly on going to bed. The spirit, wearied by the day's events might be tempted to leave too soon in the process and may suddenly cause the mind to waken the body as if alarmed. It's rather like the parent who had tried to induce sleep in his child by the comfort of his presence and then attempting to leave the room just a bit too soon, causing the child to reawaken immediately and much to the exasperation of the parent. Alternatively, the spirit may linger or stay in the body until morning. Normally in sleep, the spirit's absence or presence in the body, makes little more difference than the absence of the driver from the car.

2

While the spirit is away from the sleeping body, its experiences may be picked up by the mind and may either complicate the mind's dreaming or cause it to dream. Sometimes the spirit may transmit its experiences so clearly to the residual mind that instead of normal dreaming, the person will experience a situation which is far more real than any normal dream. Alternatively, where the spirit having left the body remains largely inactive, no particular consequence results. Where it is more active in some way, the stronger will be its signals and the greater the awareness there will be of them in the mind - resulting in the mind's dreaming being distracted or confused. It's rather like trying to think while some television plays intrusively distracting your concentration. During this more heightened active state of the spirit, it may travel to some place concerning it or the mind, say back to the workplace or some previous abode or situation. It may travel to some place to be physically visited in the future. In this latter case, giving rise to a person who subsequently actually carries out that visit, finding the place familiar and as if he feels sure he has been there before as indeed his spirit has. Where other spirits become acutely involved with the sleeping body's spirit, the very real experience of being with someone will result in what passes for an extraordinarily vivid dream.

At times the second spirit might even be the one of a deceased person. This occurs because the spirit of a 'deceased' person is almost no different to the spirit of the living and it can be encountered by the out of body spirit of the sleeper. Many people have such experiences and above all other dream experiences, this kind tend to stick in the wakened mind of the dreamer sometimes for years and even for ever.

Since the spirit is more of an intelligent charge force, and not a physical entity, it can not only move at the speed of thought from one place to the next but can also pass through any physical

3

structure too. The spirit doesn't require open doors or windows to leave the sleeper's abode nor does it need any sustenance to survive and that includes oxygen, foodstuffs, liquids or any other. Although, given time in the deceased, its energy will eventually run down and in the living, the spirit will be recharged by returning to the body. Should the spirit of the sleeping person return to the body too hurriedly, the person may awake with a jolt or experience a falling feeling just before awakening. Following decease, the spirit may not only be greatly confused by the new situation but be terribly concerned with loved ones that can no longer be physically contacted. The deceased's spirit is initially confused since the spirit is aware of what has happened, death, but is unable to understand or to grasp the new situation and may also be terribly concerned over the nature of the dismissal and how it came about. Conversely, it may be glad of the relief from some painful or worn out body. Great efforts are often made to contact the living. Somehow he survived and becomes desperate to pass on the good news to those he loved or befriended and to reassure them that he is 'fine', as indeed he is.

Enormous concern and 'heartache' can be caused to him by 'seeing' those dear to him grieving badly. He will initially attempt to touch and speak to them, seek to reassure them, but frustratingly to no avail. Sometimes, so intense is his emotional state that even the waking person may be sure he has 'seen' them, as in fact he may have, because it is both natural and common for the living griever to compensate for the loss of someone much loved, by bringing in a mirage-like image of the deceased, which can be experienced in one or more of the five senses, sight, sound, smell, touch or taste. The difference between the self-compensating mirage effect and actually being in the presence of and detecting the presence of the spirit of the deceased, would be difficult to distinguish for the griever. How does a spirit, without physical entity,

4

make contact possible? The most likely answer must be, by telepathic transmission!

If we return to the concept, highlighted in the chapter dealing with telepathy, we recall that telepathy is transmitted between two people or more, when concentrating on concentrating is abandoned for genuine interest or curiosity. Consequently, the telepathic transmission will follow similar rules between spirits rendering the efforts of the spirit concentrating on contacting a loved one unproductive. Sooner or later, much as if accidentally or alternatively just as telepathic signals can sometimes be almost instant, the spirit of the deceased may succeed and make contact with the person or persons most dear to them. However, only those on the same 'wavelength' of love and friendship will be able to engage in the mutually beneficial transmissions.

Many cases of such contacts have been both experienced and written about. More especially common are contacts during sleep where the person, thinking himself to be dreaming vividly, will be pleasantly surprised to see himself entering a familiar room or place (the place may be imagined or created by the mind to complete the picture or setting), only to find that the deceased is standing or sitting there in good health and as if nothing otherwise had happened. Alternatively, they may respond by rushing forward to meet the spirit of the living loved one emotionally not upset for themselves, but for the living spirit, seeking to welcome and reassure.

Sometimes they will say or indicate, that the living spirit should go back, as if the presence of the living spirit now on the same plane as that of the deceased, suggests to the deceased that the living spirit is risking losing his life by being there. Where two people had been greatly attached to each other particularly over a long time, the overriding desire to be reunited may induce, sometimes quickly, the desire and subsequent decision to close down or permanently abandon the body of the remaining live spirit, giving rise to an otherwise healthy person dying soon after the loss of a long-established partner.

While the deceased spirit might have some revengeful desire to contact those to whom he still holds a grudge or enmity, the attempted contact will fail because of the difference of 'wavelengths'.

Such desires, following failed attempts will be abandoned sooner rather than later. In the telepathic transmission that occurs between consenting spirits, it is as if the eyes change from cameras to become projectors and it is this combined experience of camera to projector, and consent of contact, which will enable one spirit, whether in the waking or sleeping state, to be aware of the other whilst other people present may not. As in the Bible, where some said they saw Jesus, after the crucifixion, and others with them did not. I don't say it was so, but put it forward, as a possible explanation if it was.

The following two cases illustrate this last point:

The Anxious Visiting Friend

A man called Andrew, while sitting in his front room saw his best friend coming up the path and looking terribly concerned. As Andrew got up to receive him, wondering at the reason for the unexpected visit, waved to his friend as he passed the window to ring the door bell. The door bell wasn't rung so Andrew assumed his friend saw him, rise and wave to greet him and then waited at the door. Andrew opened the door only to find nobody there and greatly curious went out to look for him but could not find him. His friend's car was not to be seen or heard leaving and yet his friend could only have come by car. Greatly mystified, he put it down to his own imaginative mind but shortly afterwards he discovered that his friend had died, earlier that same day in a terrible car accident.

The Blond Corporal

In another case, during the Second World War, a local commanding officer was amazed to see an army lorry weaving its way safely through a desert minefield. Alarmed and transfixed by the manoeuvring lorry which constantly threatened to trigger off a mine, the commander was amazed that the lorry came through safely. Following its eventual safe passage, the commander hurriedly approached the smiling relaxed driver. "Do you know you've just driven through a minefield?", the commander shouted. "Yes sir", said the driver, "I had every confidence in your corporal who showed us the way", replied the driver enthusiastically. "What corporal?", the commander barked agitatedly. "The blond one", said the driver - "good looking, about twenty-years-old." The commander was in a state of disbelief because he had watched the entire complicated manoeuvre and there was nobody else in sight, certainly not the corporal described by the confident driver.

It was then that an idea came to the commander who took the driver to a tent. Pulling back a blood-stained blanket from a dead corporal, the commander impatiently stated: "This is the only blond corporal that fits your description"."That's him", cried the now shocked and confused driver. "Well it can't be, he was killed this morning, hours before you arrived", barked back the commander. "It can't be so", replied the driver, "he was fit and well and he guided us in detail. There was nothing wrong with him at all". Make of these cases what you will but many similar ones have also been reported.

Relieving the Grief of the Bereaved

A deceased spirit of a mature person, seems normally to 'live' in the spiritual world for about half the time span of his preceding life although it may vary with life's satisfaction, some will be reluctant to relive while others are impatient to do so. If the spirit is from a person who was 'bad' or 'wicked' in life, in the spiritual world he will become aware of his actions and have to endure his guilt-based on the life he had led which was based upon his genetic inheritance, his own faulty self-programming, his reactions, experiences, deeds and endeavours. The spirit, now neutral of those effects suffers the anguish of his life's actions. This self-revelation may occur instantly, soon or take time. In short, he suffers his own 'hell'. Under sufficient persisting anxiety, he may remain in the spiritual state until his energy runs down completely and then he truly is deceased, irretrievably gone as it were. So too with the reluctant to return to life, having had sufficiently awful life experiences. In the case of young people, especially small children lose their life, a return to a new life can be swift.

So the question arises of how does a spirit gain the new life? It could be that at a time of peace, when the spirit has recovered from life's experiences, the spirit will take up the occupation of an unborn foetus and in this way, reincarnation occurs. Going back to the original 'mechanical' or physiological process of conception to birth, we can start to unravel the path.

First there is the production of spermatozoa and although physically active, it cannot be claimed to be a complete human being so therefore, most unlikely to have its own spirit, for the spirit enters from the combination of what makes us human. Next we have the female egg. This, in the same way, cannot be seen as a complete human either. When both egg and sperm combine, it can be argued that still no human exists, for the cells need to divide, grow and develop, to form special parts of the forming body or foetus. I hold that not until the process is sufficiently advanced, will a spirit take up residence, and that time is likely to be around five, six or seven months into gestation. Consequently in cases of an early miscarriage or abortion, some hope of consolation can be given to the mother because where no human spirit exists no real human does either. In some cases, a woman who has suffered a miscarriage, or undergone an abortion will have terrible feelings of guilt, anger or remorse.//As a result she may feel, on giving birth following a subsequent pregnancy, that child is difficult to love, perhaps seeming to her to be a second-class baby in some way whereas in reality, the spirit or essence of that subsequent child could well have been the spirit of the earlier pregnancy//It is rather as if the child has made it at the second attempt and as such, deserves greater welcome and love rather than less. Even if there is only a one percent chance of the process put forward being right, with the subjects acceptance of the principle, sufficient positive doubt will exist, to greatly ease the lot of the mother who had lost a previous foetus. The greater the acceptance of such a possibility, the greater it will help her, even to the extent of entirely freeing the mother to enjoy a far happier experience, in dealing with and loving her child, by the sheer wonder of it all.

When dealing with a grief-stricken bereaved, with caution, I put forward what I consider appropriate from the above. When I have, I ask if they think it's possible, even remotely so, and if there just might be some truth in what has been said. If you proceed with the explanations above with care, tact and kindness, interrupting your progress by enquiring if the subject is coping with what's being put forward, then most will agree, that there is at least some possibility that it could have some truth in it. To further assist in relieving a grieving client I tactfully, having welcomed their positive response, proceed to ask of them for whom they cry, or cried (or feel sorry for) in their loss. Eventually, if not immediately, with similar gentle encouragement, they will stumble upon the great truth that, at base, their sorrow or grief is for themselves, in their sense of loss. Of course, there can be nothing wrong in this natural sense of self-pity at all. Having got them to realise it, you can proceed, checking your progress as you go, such as by asking if they are coping and handling it or by seeking their reassurance that you are not pushing them too far. By doing so, if they find it too much for them in some way, you give them a chance to say so. If they feel under pressure, you must decide on whether to encourage them, by suggesting that there's not much more to come, 'back off' or suggest that you (we) might return to it at another time when the client has had time to consider it more.

Since the preceding process is always carried out in hypnosis, even where doubt of its truth is high, sufficient acceptance will remain of its reassuring possibility to help them recover from the grief anyway. Either in continuing or returning to the subject later, I go on to remind them that their grief is primarily and naturally for themselves which is entirely and fully understandable. I then suggest that if what has been said was even remotely possibly true, it must also equally be possibly true that the lost loved one, drawn by the occasion (the now) could be in spiritual form and unseen, present in the room. Having come so far, it is only logical that they should agree at least to the possibility.

Again with caution, tact, empathy and understanding, I ask them to imagine the departed and how they must feel, knowing how upset you (the subject) are (or have been). "They can't hug you, speak to you; tell you they are okay; they can't wipe your tears (if the client is crying as mostly they will be); they can't cheer you up or reassure you". "They're all right but can't pass you that message". "In fact, the only thing they are suffering from is seeing you, the one they so loved (or liked) in the unhappy state you are

10

in" (or have been in). "Tell me", I ask at a carefully chosen point, "if what I say is true but the situation was reversed, that is you were in the room looking on and it was your loved one (or friend) in the chair, what would you want them to do?" With some gentle encouragement they respond along the lines that they would want them to cheer up and get on with life and to stop feeling sad. This reaction can then be reinforced by such suggestions as: "So the hurt would go". "So that the love (friendship) can go on in a worthwhile sense without sorrow detracting from it". "They can show that the love (friendship) was worthwhile by delighting you with how well they get on with life so that the love (friendship) can continue in a rewarding way".

In most cases the client will readily agree that such a response would be much more desirable to them and they wouldn't want their loved one (friend) to be upset over them. After a short pause and in a firmer measured tone, tinged with an element of emotion I then say: "Then why not take your own advice?" This can be followed with a more light-hearted discussion covering aspects of the deceased or what has just been discussed and what the client could now go on to do, etc. Expect much improvement in your previously grieving client to follow shortly.

Sometimes, the reincarnation principle put forward can also have other uses. Around their early thirties many for the first time, confront themselves with the prospect of eventually dying, sometimes with devastating emotional effects and with some even becoming almost obsessed with the idea. Using the principle given, great relief can be expected here too.

Personally in such cases, I put the concept forward in a far more light-hearted, reassuring manner than the sympathetic caution to be adopted with the bereaved. Highlighting the benefits of the process of renewal, eternity and indestructibility. After putting across the principle and having their agreement that it could be

11

possible some of the suggestions I might make, depending on whether the client is male or female, include the following examples. For instance, I may ask them if the car they have now is the last one they could have, what condition would it be in say in 50 or 60 years time, long before then they would want to replace it wouldn't they? Well, isn't it also better, to have a new body too from time to time? Think of the state you would be in, in a thousand years from now? No, nature has a much better scheme, and in this way you live on for ever, by being given a new body from time to time, you get a fresh start. That way you can be here in a thousand years time just as you may have been here a thousand years ago but with a healthy and fit body. It's all rather reassuring that nature never commits so many resources to life to see it all wasted. I often smile or laugh by saying I call it '*just going round again*'.

Sometimes, I might give the example of my Service days or illustrate the educational process. In the former I say how strange it was at my first posting. At first I knew nobody; didn't know my way about the camp or the local rules; who was who; what to watch out for; what opportunities existed or could be created. Everyone on camp would be wiser than me.

Gradually things would change as I gained friends and learnt from experience until I became one of the longest serving members on the camp and then much wiser, seeing new intakes arriving and feeling lost and seeking the advice I had once sought. Just about that time I would find myself posted on again. Although wiser then, I'd still find myself a greenhorn at my new posting and the process experienced in the earlier posting, would be just the same but quicker. With posting following posting, on each occasion there would be both regrets at leaving and new adventures to be experienced in arriving. All-in-all, it was a wonderful part of my life.

Life-to-life experiences could be viewed in much the same way for we also gradually evolve too. Again, everyone has the experience of going through their school years, starting with play school, then nursery school, junior school, senior school and college or university. Each is a stage in life not the life itself.

In a further comparison I often put forward another way that life cycles could be viewed, in this the client is asked to compare a life span to the length of a long day. Just as we may tire from a sixteen-to-eighteen-hour day and then go to bed to recuperate and awaken refreshed for the new day, so one life to another can be imagined.

Generally speaking, a spirit returning to take up the occupancy of a foetus will select not only the same sex as previously experienced, preferring as it were the familiar, but also a similar family type that they had been accustomed to in their previous life. It is as if they are once again drawn back to their earlier roots. Together with the inherited genetics, family attitudes and early life experiences this produces some family tendencies like going into law, the armed forces, the medical world, becoming academically adept or taking up some other lifestyle. For example, if in a previous life we had done well in some field or had a considerable interest in something, then on rebirth we might well carry that inclination forward. Now we might have the gifted artist in the family that is inartistic or a fairly ordinary family may find in their offspring, a gifted mathematician, doctor, engineer or aspiring in some other way.

Although complications might arise should a change in sex occur from one life to the next. Further 'evidence' of rebirth can occur in other ways such as the near blind child painting pictures of things he could never have seen, or the child that develops to have almost nothing but his looks and appearance in common with his family.

In this last case, the returning spirit has most likely and for some reason, accidentally 'changed places' as it were rather like the 'stork' delivering the baby to the 'wrong' home. There could be

13

reasons for this too. In a former life for instance, a distaste of his experiences may lead to a change of desire and cause him to seek an alternative existence, or the spirit ready to return to life, being beaten to its intended foetus by another spirit with similar needs. The person, having ended his days in some other part of the world, may linger there spiritually becoming reborn as a native. There may be the desire to return to a previous life's environment but if the previous environment no longer exists it cannot do so.

Mostly however, the spirit will seek to return to familiar settings. If the concept of renewal through reincarnation is accepted, and it widely is, there comes a possibility that we become our own great or great-great-grandchildren. Before the spirit takes up its occupation of the foetus, several visits are normally made, like visits by a purchaser to a house being built. Although in this case, occupation takes place prior to completion, i.e, before birth.

Past Lives Regression

Another use of the reincarnation theory is in dealing with past life experiences. However, it's rare in my experience for a client to approach me feeling they might be affected by a previous life. Where clients do ask for regression therapy from curiosity, I usually dissuade them. Unless something really significant has happened to them in a previous life, it will mean several visits with their experiences often proving uneventful for the client and possibly boring to the therapist. This is because mostly only fairly ordinary lives are experienced and it may take several uneventful sessions, in which only vague unconnected impressions emerge. However, it is essential in a regression of this kind that the therapist should do nothing to put any suggestion into the client's mind. The therapist must listen, only asking questions neutrally, such as: "Is anyone with you?" rather than, "who else is there?", or "what happens next?", rather than, "does so and so happen?", etc. Even such carefully framed questions can carry suggestions and lead to a wild-goose chase. If regression is carried out properly, it requires great patience by both client and therapist alike. Personally, I feel I have more important healing work to do and would leave curiosity regression to others more suited to its demands.

From time-to-time, particularly with left-brain types, reincarnation will be dismissed out of hand as bunkum with such people possibly asking the therapist if he ever saw a dead body. In doing so, he is making the assumption that reincarnation is the coming back to life of the body. He may consider that the concept of reincarnation is due to excessive and ridiculous imagination, dreamt up by someone on the verge of some awful psychosis. Except that in turn, he doesn't accept that the psychotic state is anything but a person failing to pull himself together. With anything like a rejection of this kind, I would advise the reader to drop the matter quickly. One day he is in for an enormously confusing surprise and a great revelation.

At my own mother's funeral service I listened incredulously to the clergyman attempting to put forward a concept of rising from the grave. He did so by explaining the process as coming back to the surface through the action of bacteria, microbes, worms and insects so that the person becomes the substance of the grass, trees and flowers and in this way, is reincarnated to become the great beauty of the world around us. I doubt that his concept was accepted by anyone in the congregation and yet the concept of the spirit, as a separate part of us, is a consistent theme of most religions. I sometimes think that the church would be more respected if it concentrated more on what many consider to be the true spiritual nature of humans. For instance, some people, and in one case even a Bishop of the Church of England, dismiss the concept of Christ being born of the virgin Mary, saying that a birth to a virgin is unthinkable. Yet using the theory set out, would it not have been possible for the spirit of Jesus to have been that of the Son of God? If the principle is accepted, neither Joseph or Mary could have produced the spirit only the 'body'. Accepting that possibility Mary, the Mother of Jesus, didn't have to be a 'pure' virgin for Jesus, the Son of God to be born.

So the argument over the issue fades away and the concept becomes realistic and understandable I wonder too, how many more people, by knowing that reincarnation actually happens would seek to improve their lives and attend church more often? If the church rid itself of some of its man-made interpretations and concentrated on the true spiritual aspects and thereby help people to appreciate the great wonder of it all, I suspect that people would flock to it. Some religions subscribe to the theory that, in reincarnation, we progress spiritually from the smallest living organisms to the human stage. While there is no proof of this progression, there's no proof that is could not be so. Since it seems overwhelmingly the case that we even reappear as the same sex, I find it a difficult theory to accept, that we animals and creatures, can somehow have 'interchangeable' spirits in reincarnation, seems most unlikely.

A further point of interest is the possibility of a human having been reduced physically, mentally or both to such a low state that the spirit, suffering the disharmony, may wish to 'escape' from that living person as much as possible. Where this condition is reached, that spirit may try to enter the body of another person less badly affected whose spirit has also developed the preference of absence. In such a case the person becomes or feels possessed, or suffers a spiritual conflict of body ownership. As the more disturbed spirit is more determined and will carry with it some sense of its original body and mind, the possessed may react in extraordinary ways and quite out of their normal character.

When the possessed is psychologically strengthened during analysis, by removing their malaise, the spirit of the former possessed person is not only now stronger but more willingly residential. Conversely, having left the body it can return more determinedly should such a subsequent invasion threaten, the unhappy spirit of the other person then looking elsewhere for an easier target.

Treatment of the possessed can be difficult because two powerful but separate conditions can exist. Firstly, there is the condition that led to the reduced circumstances of the victim which made him vulnerable. Secondly, the invading spirit or even spirits will do all that is possible to cling to the new possession by attempting to produce resistance; to force the victim into non-cooperation to treatment. In this, the church may be of considerable help since some church members have developed great skills in this area. Fortunately, possession of this kind is rare and may be ignored by the vast majority of therapists and is only mentioned, so as not to leave a potentially important area out of consideration.

✳Another important aspect of reincarnation, previously touched upon but warranting a more specific consideration, is what might be called 'decisive recycling'. To understand this process we must remind ourselves once again, that the mind runs the body, that the subconscious lacks intelligence but carries out what it understands to be the command of the programme and without querying it; and that the subconscious is aware of reincarnation.✳

In decisive recycling we can have the situation in which the subconscious concludes that this life should be discontinued and another begun. This conclusion or decision, once becoming part of the programme, will then be run if uninterrupted or unchanged until the objective is attained. The fundamental reasons for selecting that objective can be many and varied. When this principle was

17

introduced earlier, it was illustrated by the surviving member of a partnership terminating life, so that the body's spirit could permanently regain that partnership and join the deceased partner permanently, on the same spiritual plane. However, many other factors can contribute to a decisive recycling decision. A person may become totally weary of life, either physically mentally or both. They may suffer, perhaps without realising it at a conscious level, tremendous feelings of guilt, uselessness, pessimism, self-hate, depression or any other strong emotion leaving the subconscious to conclude that only by quitting or leaving life, can they escape that life's awfulness. Such a decision can take many routes to its fulfilment. It may disable some vital part, suddenly or slowly. It may induce suicide or cause an indifference to risk, leaving others to observe that the victim has a 'death wish'.

Where one process is interrupted, another begins yet sometimes the reaction itself can be the cry for help, the subconscious being aware of the conflict between self-preservation and self-destruction. This is noticeable in failed suicide attempts or where the suicidal suddenly calls for help having taken some substance or action which has not yet had its otherwise intended effect. Two cases of decisive recycling serve to illustrate the principle. Note: it is only by happenstance that both were female clients.

The Lady Smoking Herself to Death

A lady attended for anti-smoking therapy, and gave as her motivating reason the fact that her father had died of lung cancer which was attributed to his smoking. This was a profound loss to her so she didn't want her children to face the same prospect of losing her. As you will find, should you use it, the anti-smoking therapy to be given is highly effective, even for those remotely interested in quitting. However, the day following her session she reported that it had absolutely no effect. Curious as to why, I invited the lady to re-attend and when she did, I asked her subconscious to tell her conscious mind what purpose her smoking served that was causing it to override the benefits of becoming a non-smoker. With tears then rolling down her face and in great surprise, she informed me her subconscious had said smoking was being used to terminate her life; that she was to smoke herself to death just as her father had done. In short, her conscious mind wanted to survive but unknown to her, her subconscious did not.

On probing further, the lady revealed that she had a disastrous marriage, being the victim of extreme mental sadistic cruelty from her husband, even though he acted in a most caring, considerate manner towards her in public and in company. Good looking, intelligent and charming, he was fooling everyone into thinking his wife was just imagining her allegations of cruelty. He was leading them to think she was simply neurotic and that he, the kind, considerate and attentive caring husband was coping with his undeserving wife with exceptional understanding, tolerance and fortitude.

The reality was that alone at home, he took great delight in endlessly mentally torturing her. Set against outward appearances and the absence of any sign of physical harm, she was experiencing great difficulty in pursuing her petition for divorce and obtaining a local authority house for herself and her two children. In her near impossible situation, she couldn't leave because she had nowhere else to go. Fortunately, a factor not taken into account by her subconscious was that she had by then, almost reached her goal of being offered a home. By psychologically building her up, she was able to reduce her smoking and able to quit altogether, a few months after moving in to her new home which she eventually obtained.

The Lady with Eight Weeks to Live

In the second case, a lady reported that she had been given, on Boxing Day morning, the news that she had a maximum of eight weeks to live, her medical condition being too far advanced to respond to any further treatment - a battle of five years having been lost. I'm being deliberately vague as to the nature of her condition in order to avoid raising hopes in others who may be similarly affected. I would rather report what happened in her case by way of illustrating the decisive recycling principle. The lady in question did not come for the treatment of her condition but rather for assistance with dying with dignity. (Perhaps a last minute cry for help?) As can be done, and as is also described later it is possible, with suitable co-operation, to have the subconscious speak directly, that is for it to take the voice over. This was successfully carried out. In hypnosis, let's call her Jan, here's how the exchange proceeded.

Therapist: "Subconscious have you caused this condition to come into being for some purpose?"

Client: "Yes".

Therapist: "Subconscious, if you thought it more appropriate to do so, could you send Jan's condition into remission, completely totally and permanently?"

Client: "Yes".

Therapist: "Then, subconscious, why have you caused this condition to come into being?"

Client: "Because Jan is unhappy, nasty, big-headed, and deserves to die".

Therapist: "Thank you subconscious. Subconscious, if I could suggest a better way of looking after Jan, would you be prepared to consider it?"

Client:	"Yes!"
Therapist:	"Subconscious, to make such a suggestion, I need to know and understand Jan better, this will take time, would you agree to commence the remission process, to give me the time I require?"
Client:	"Yes!"
Therapist:	"Then subconscious, when I count to three, and click my fingers, please make the changes needed to commence the remission".

On the *click* the lady opened her eyes reporting that a sudden shock had gone through her entire body. During the six weeks of analysis, she continued to make progress with her condition, and her subconscious anxiety being resolved resulted in her condition being released. Following analysis, a subsequent plan calling for a far more fulfilling and satisfying life was put forward and accepted by her subconscious. On May 31st and some five months later, she was contacted to enquire of her progress. Amazingly it took several seconds for her to recall who we were, but then stated life to be 'fine' and reported she had virtually forgotten the matter.

In talking of spiritual matters from time-to-time, the accusation of dealing or dabbling in the paranormal is made. My response to such allegations, where the accuser will listen, is that there can be no paranormal for the term is in itself contradictory, intending to mean another or alternative normality one somehow running side-by-side with 'normal' normality, as if there was a gap in the laws covering normality that allowed other laws to coincide, or even to be random in nature or be 'magical' as if there could be exceptions to everything else, as if there could also be paranormal gravity, paranormal chemistry or mathematics. That which is called paranormal is just a name and no more than that, for labelling that which is simply not yet understood. Paranormal is an all-embracing term used by those who cannot, will not, or have not really considered the question seriously. In the concept that this term is used, it implies that the unexplained and mysterious must be the result of some chaotic exception to the natural laws of nature and reality. In such 'reasoning' we cut ourselves off from the logic, science and enquiry we need to progress. Or is the name and what it implies a convenient excuse not to look deeper and probe, for like the giant silver bird (the aircraft) ignorance makes the unaccounted for, seem spooky, mystifying and forbidding.

Years ago, in Africa, aircraft were regarded as 'paranormal' and often much dreaded. In some parts of the world you might even have been killed by the natives if you attempted to take their photograph for in doing so, you were thought of by them as capturing their spirit and in this sense, the camera was a paranormal device. As human skills and knowledge increase, that which is 'magical', 'paranormal' or 'mysterious' becomes increasingly understood and each example is found, in turn, to fit precisely into the natural order of things.

Take radio and television for instance, if you had no knowledge of them at all and someone set out to suggest that thousands of invisible radio signals were travelling through the air at the speed of light, often spanning the world and that in such signals were voices, sounds and pictures, you might think of them as insane. Or conversely, you might go outside to listen or look but all to no avail. If it were then said that these signals travel down an 'aerial' and into a 'box' so that you can hear and see them, would you believe them? No, although you might be generous and just consider them eccentric. Should such a 'box' or set be switched on you might become alarmed at the inexplicable result. To you this would be the paranormal. Now imagine going to a friend to tell him of your experience - a friend who also knows nothing of such things? As with this radio and television example, even those who are open-minded but with no known experience of the spiritual concept, can find that concept of reincarnation and the spirit difficult to accept. This is mostly because they have never consciously encountered a situation that would have brought them to the point where awareness could have occurred. However, once aware, further occasions will normally be experienced.

The Case of the Absent Driver

In one case a man reported to me he'd been caught up in congested high-speed traffic, just after the motorway he was travelling on had merged with another. He found himself in the midst of the traffic unable to overtake or pull into the left, a tightly-bunched column of vehicles near to his rear and he was too close behind the lorry in front. He was tired having had a stressful day. He just knew there was going to be a terrible accident. Suddenly he found himself in the air, travelling just over the rear of his car. He could see himself driving as if the car's roof was made of glass but could feel nothing but could see his hands on the steering wheel with no sensation of touch - it was as if he was watching somebody else but knew it was himself.

After travelling some distance the traffic began to space itself out more and he suddenly found himself back as the driver. By then he was near to home and concluded his journey safely. Following this experience he was horrified to find that what he disregarded as imagination brought on by his stress, began to recur gradually more and more frequently but only on motorways. The experiences eventually reduced him to using only the slow lane. "Now", he reported, "I can even experience it on the approach slipway and it's impossible for me to go on with my job which calls for a lot of driving". In going back to the original event, together with finding the underlying cause of the stress he had suffered for many years, he was able to restore his confidence and drive normally.

Many cases of the spirit leaving the body have been reported and are known as '*out of body experiences*' (OBEs) and are far more common than is generally realised. In addition to this, everyone continually has the experience, but most do not recognise it or realise it consciously. During operations, in emergencies or sufficiently threatening circumstances, the spirit will leave or 'escape' just as a pilot might consciously wish to eject from a crashing aeroplane. However, as it was in the previously quoted case, when the spirit leaves in a sense of opting out, it can produce an unnerving, though not dangerous consequence. In some cases, people can develop their ability to have out-of-body experiences at will. Techniques for doing so can be found in specialist books and are omitted here, since it plays no part in our work as healers being more of another matter the therapist should be aware of, albeit an intriguing one.

Personal Experiences

At the age of eight I was brutally beaten by the master of the children's home in which I was placed. The beating was intense and took place in a field where we were on a camping holiday, I suddenly found myself about twenty feet in the air, looking down on myself. The sensation was as if I was surrounded by a strong static electrical field. I could neither feel the beating nor did I feel concerned. I was instead, only curious as to what was happening. It felt lovely, a truly peaceful feeling of detachment. Suddenly I was brought back into my body as it was dragged away by nurses from the protesting master. Then it was that I felt the awful pain.

In the six months I was in the home, my mother found

another partner. One day, seemingly out of the blue I was collected by a staff member of the home and taken into a room where, to my amazement and delight, my mother greeted me. She told me her news and that she had come to collect me. I hastily gathered my few possessions together and eagerly listened as my mother described her new partner and the house in which I was to live. Naturally, on arriving at the new house, everything seemed strange at first but as the young can, I soon settled down.

A few days later, asleep in my bed, I was gradually awoken in response to a gentle tapping on my door. I sat up in the darkness and invited the person knocking to come in. The door didn't open but the knocking continued. After two or three similar invitations and by then fully awake, I climbed out of my bed and opened the door. I was surprised to find a beautiful girl of about eleven or twelve years of age standing there smiling at me. I can't remember exactly what I said but it was probably along the lines of "Yes!" or "What do you want?" or similar.

The girl just kept looking at me and smiling as she did, I firstly became mystified then vaguely apprehensive. As I did, I began to realise I could see through her, details of the landing behind her. My apprehensiveness suddenly turned to great alarm because I didn't understand it but realised something very strange was taking place. Suddenly I slammed the door in her face and cried out as I ran back to my bed. I pulled the bed clothes over me and lay there trembling with my heart racing.

Somehow I eventually fell asleep. All this could have been dismissed as imagination or some dream or nightmare but for what happened the following morning. At the breakfast table, my mother angrily asked if it had been me who slammed a door in the night and shouted out waking everyone. When I confessed she demanded an explanation which I gave, whereupon my newly-acquired stepfather demanded a description of the girl.

As I gave it by describing her in a red dressing gown, pageboy hairstyle, build, height and round face, he turned white, dropped his knife and fork and left the table in considerable distress. My mother was alarmed and asked him why he had reacted as he did. While looking at me in a rather menacing accusative way, as he pointed his finger at me, he exclaimed: "He's just described Junie in detail". "Who's Junie?", mother asked. "Who?", he replied, "she was a distant relative who died of pneumonia in this house ten years ago".

Two weeks later, my younger brother had a similar encounter. The innocent spirit merely came to meet us, meaning nothing more serious than that. However for my part, for some 40 years I would suffer attacks of migraine that always came on around one o'clock in the night and while I was asleep. It was an unusual case of migraine and one that baffled the doctors. I never connected that night's experience to my migraine until during my analysis I was to come across that memory again. I am happy to report, this time for myself, the migraine has been gone for years.

Two further personal experiences are worth recording. During the advanced stages of my wife's last pregnancy, I awoke in the early hours of the night on three occasions, to find two very clear beautiful spirits in the room. Only the head and shoulders of each were visible, but both were at a height they would naturally have been as standing adults. Knowing what I did by then, I was free, for the few seconds they remained on each occasion, to be able to enjoy the experiences. I became convinced that despite what we then thought to be the case of my wife expecting a single child, she was to have twins. It was of course, the spiritual visits made before foetal occupation was taken up, as referred to earlier. Since the spirits were visibly female, I happily looked forward to the arrival of twin daughters.

On the third occasion, I was awoken once again to see

those same two spirits but this time, only their faces were visible, and just a few inches above my wife's midriff. Suddenly as I watched, both disappeared and I remain convinced at that moment, foetal occupation was taken up. About ten weeks later, my daughter duly arrived, healthy and well. Why only one child? I believe that much as we would prefer to be accompanied in life on all important occasions, and as much as we are greeted on leaving life by a fellow kindred spirit, we are accompanied as we prepare to enter life again.

If what I strongly hold to be the case, based upon my own experiences and what I have read, the hundreds of examples that have been given to me by clients are true, then far from any spookiness it is an exciting, reassuring process. It means not only that we live on and survive our dismissals but those loved ones that precede us are not lost in some ghastly final act either. All in all, a process that is greatly to be welcomed.

On Suicide

Before closing this chapter in which far more could be said, I feel the subject of suicide must be considered. Anyone who commits suicide finds to their cost, as several clients have come to realise, where past life experiences have intruded into this life, suicide is never a solution but rather an extension to their problem. The emotion which leads to the act, continues to be felt in the spiritual plane but by then, the person will lack the physical ability to take any action to resolve their plight. Added to this is the misery of seeing those left behind, in dreadfully reduced states and often for the rest of their lives.

I think that its this terrible combination that makes even meeting on the spiritual plane of those who have committed suicide, far less frequent than would normally be the case. In short, the exasperations of life are compounded by guilt, shame, sadness and emotional pain. The person seeing themselves the victim of life becomes the unforgivable victim of themselves - even in cases of subsequent rebirth, where regression becomes necessary to resolve a problem that has spilled into this life, the tragic end of a former life that has never been forgotten or finally resolved.

The Lonely Man

In one case a man in his early twenties reported to me that he was utterly unable to have any real bond with anyone. As a boy he distanced himself even from his parents and brothers, always tried to be alone at school and stood in the corner of the playground at playtimes. He was never able to take up the invitations of would-be friends and added that, although wishing he could mix with others, he would feel so self-conscious, so ill-at-ease and uncomfortable that he would feel compelled to withdraw from any 'threat' of company. He readily agreed that it was not their fault and when on his own he felt a strange feeling of even wanting to walk away from himself. He had felt, in some mysterious way, a sense of awfulness all of his life and would often burst into tears for no explicable reason.

Now he'd met a girl and wanted the relationship to flourish, but he kept their meetings as infrequent and as brief as possible. This inner 'thing' was making his attempt to develop the relationship not only impossible but likely soon to destroy it. If they were out together he wanted her to walk on in front. To hold hands with her took enormous self-determination. When he drove her in the car, he insisted she sit in the back "for safety reasons". On his fourth visit, I asked him if he came to his sessions by car, to which he replied: "Yes". I pointed out to him that in the area it was often difficult to park, so he could use the forecourt kept clear for client's convenience. He said he couldn't do that because his car, being several hundred yards away, meant as he saw it, that he was at least keeping himself in part, away from me like an act of dissociation or incomplete contact. "Sometimes I feel suicidal but when I do think of it I will be physically sick", he reported on one occasion.

The sessions continued until the eighth was halfway through but still with no signs of change or improvement of any kind and with nothing tangible having come to light. During the second-half of the session I decided to ask his subconscious if it would confirm that his problem had stemmed from this life's experiences. His subconscious responded by saying that it didn't. It was then asked if the problem stemmed from some experiences while still in the womb with "No" being the response. "Does the problem originate from a former life's experience", I asked his subconscious, and to this his subconscious answered, somewhat vigorously: "Yes!" and the man instantly became highly emotional.

When his subconscious was asked to go back to that former life's experiences, in a state of even greater emotion he saw himself jump from a tall building and fall to his death. He then began to recall being aware of, and seeing grieving friends and relatives. Banging the arms of the chair in which he sat in anguish, he reported that, in a state of remorse for his actions he had repeatedly attempted to express his sorrow for his selfish action, "But they ignore me, it's as if I'm not there".

Then he suddenly shouted out: "It's her - I see it now, I've had a row with my girlfriend, we're finished she says ... oh God, it was only a row, oh God! oh God!" The client was becoming exhausted and by now had cried so much, that the front of his shirt was soaking wet, despite my attempts to mop his tears as they came. Gradually, over the next half-hour or so he regained his composure, but even after a nearly two hour long session left with tears still in his eyes.

I was surprised when he next arrived because for the first time, he drove straight onto my forecourt and surprise, surprise, from the passenger seat out stepped his girlfriend whom I was to meet for the very first time. He was brimming with enthusiasm and she had come to express her gratitude. Enthusiastically he poured out the events of his life over the last few days and he couldn't believe the difference he had found in himself. He said he had applied to become a Samaritan. "Nobody's better qualified to talk to suicidals more than me", he said.

Just before he left he added: "By the way, I haven't had my nightmare this week". "What nightmare?" I asked. "Well", he said, "I used to have a nightmare, once or twice a week in which I'd suddenly find myself on a cliff top looking out to sea. After a few moments, a great gust of wind would blow me over the edge, and I'd watch myself fall to my death on the rocks below".

"I asked you if you had nightmares, and you said no", I responded. "Ah yes, they were so hideous that I could never have talked about them to anyone - anyway, I didn't see any connection with them and my problem".

Chapter Two

The Oedipus and Electra Complexes

Of all the chapters in this series of books, this one has proved to be the most difficult, not because of any lack of knowledge or experience of the subject, nor because there are several equally good ways of presenting it with each competing with the other, but rather because the concept and subject itself can be objectionable to some. In practice I find this objection, despite every effort to be tactful and even with audiences where its inclusion is appropriate as a subject. The subject however has been referred to before in these writings, by way of an introduction.

I always make a point of including the treatment of these complexes with every client coming to me for analysis and I am mindful that my treatment success rate, as judged by the clients themselves, is higher than I have ever heard any other therapist claiming. This is not to say that no therapist does as well or even better, but rather that I have not yet met or heard of one that has made a superior claim. Furthermore, could it be a coincidence that I am also the only therapist I know of, who does routinely cover the complexes with clients?

If I seem to be labouring on the subject or stand to risk the accusation of boasting, I hope that I am not, for the points are only put forward as an introduction to the two complexes and to help stress the immensity of their importance as a subject.

Following the failed attempts of analysis with four other therapists, I eventually went through analysis successfully with a very talented and experienced female therapist, losing both my migraine and panic-attack problems as I did so. However, on a subsequent occasion with my wife as the therapist, I decided to take my own advice and check for the presence, in myself of the Oedipus complex, since this had not been specifically included in my analysis. Bingo, for over three weeks I had a feeling of release, even elevation that I was almost constantly aware of. There could be no doubt but that I was a victim of the condition myself. Yet in attempting to put the issue forward to one tutor I was effectively told that it was merely 'Freudian bunkum'.

In another case, a hypnotherapist accused me of being obsessed with the complexes and declined to consider them for treatment. In the analysis he conducted for both my wife and I, there was no beneficial effect for either of us. Not only this, but in all of the fifteen other people I have met who went through analysis with the same hypnotherapist, all reported the same negative outcome. When comparing this with the success rate I find, by using the methods given in this series of books, of over ninety percent the case for including the complexes as a standard practice in therapy appears overwhelming.

In the thousands of clients who consulted me, the relevant complex has proved to be the single most common foundation for their neurotic conditions. When this is added to the seemingly endless range of symptoms the complexes can produce, and then go on to further add the awfulness that these symptoms can bring, it becomes difficult to see how the importance of the subject could be over-stressed. Significantly, in the session following the one in which these complexes are discussed, I find some sixty percent of clients reporting major improvements in how they are then feeling.

In my opinion, only three reasons can exist for omitting these two vital complexes in therapy. Firstly, since they can produce such widespread and enormous subconscious anxiety, some hypnotherapists can be suspected, at least in part, to have been drawn to the profession by them. In which case, as a further defence of their own repressions of them, the concept itself must be denied. This attitude is further underscored, by those who ridicule Freud, who despite whatever he may be accused of, was a founder of the analysis concept and is still the most widely known in the entire history of analytical practice. Secondly, probably flowing from the first reason, the two complexes seem hardly to be taught, at least as far as I understand it when speaking to the therapists that I have met from several different training colleges. Certainly they are not commonly taught as treatment methods.

One glaring exception to this is the Neil French school of hypnotherapy based in Bournemouth. Thirdly, the complexes are the consequences of the internally repressed group, producing direct, indirect and contrived symptoms, and because of this, they can be reflected in any of the physiological, psychological and behavioural ways, and identifying them may at first seem over complicated or too difficult although (as will be shown) no such problems actually exist. Despite the simplicity of resolving them, perhaps the greatest stumbling block, for some hypnotherapists is the one given in chapter 6, Book One, explaining the internally repressed event. That is, too frequently the method of how to resolve such repressions is simply not known! To qualify that viewpoint I have in my possession a letter from a prominent member of the profession who is himself an examiner of hypnotherapists, asking how to do it! Fortunately, by simply reading this work, none of those 'problems' need apply.

Now to tackle that difficult question of setting it out, but before doing so I ask you keep an open mind. Males are observed to have the ability to create an erection in less than an hour from birth. This demonstrates firstly, sex is present from birth and secondly, that sex must be under the control of the subconscious: for it would be absurd to think that an infant, at such an early stage, could be consciously or intelligently be sufficiently aware to respond in this way. Thirdly, it demonstrates, not only the cleverness of the subconscious to be able to create that response, but also that that part of the mind lacks intelligence, i.e., it is able to create the erection, but is not intelligent enough to perceive the futility of doing so! Following birth, the baby boy will be brought up, certainly in his most formative years, by a woman and almost always she is his mother. Other women may play a role even a dominant one, like a nurse to an orphan, a grandmother, aunt, sister, nanny, foster-mother or some other, such as the lady next door.

However, it is a woman, or women who will play a constant attentive role in his first few years. In the case of the female infant, her sexuality is just as present as it is in the male, but of course mainly undetected. She too, is to have a female or females having a dominant role in her formative years. But in this case, and I state the obvious to emphasise the point, it will be a female-female relationship, whereas in the male infant relationship, it is a male-female one. Furthermore, there can be a situation in the female-female relationship, of the infant female with no significant male presence.

However, it is almost unimaginable for a male infant to experience only a male-male relationship. This essential difference, in our parental relationships, in our early years can have enormous consequences for us as adults. These are more beneficial as a whole, rather than negative. Where negative effects do result they can have serious consequences. Both complexes have many similarities and can produce similar symptoms and effects, consequently to avoid repetition as far as possible, it is not practical to attempt to set out a clearly separated explanation of either on its own.

The Oedipus Complex

The Oedipus Complex is named after a legendary Greek, who

married his mother without being aware of her identity. Briefly, the Oedipus Complex is the consequence of the male infant misunderstanding his true relationship with his mother believing instead, that he and his mother are partners, equally and exclusively attracted to each other and bound in a common bond. Whilst few complications result during the initial stage, many may result, as it gradually becomes realised by the infant that the relationship is a mother and son bond and therefore becomes subconsciously perceived as slipping away, in its originally held form thus leaving him to view others, particularly his father, as superior rivals and subsequently and ultimately having to confront his loss.

Using our male child example, we see that following his birth, it will normally be his mother that first feeds him by breast or bottle. At this time of enormous satisfaction, following the trauma of his birth, he gazes into his mother's face. Over the months ahead, he will increasingly come to see in that face, a reassuringly familiar sight, a welcome, lovely sight. His subconscious will also sense her to be a female, attractive and different to him and result in subconscious sexual reactions sooner or later. The mother will most likely see these subconscious sexual reactions because they will be displayed eventually in a physical manner. The erections which result are sexual in origin and not physiological accidents.

I once had a male client who was an orphan but sadly, his nurse had amused herself by taking advantage of his sexual reactions to her 'care' by masturbating him. Although there could be no ejaculation, the client clearly remembered the sexual excitement it gave him. He was a victim of this sexual abuse, from the age of eighteen months, with the experiences occurring for some time and until the nurse left the orphanage. The combined effect of these early sexual experiences and the sudden loss of his mother figure, were to have disastrous effects on his life not least, in that he could never trust a woman again and remained single. If not for this mistrust that resulted from her activities, in my opinion, he would have made an excellent, understanding husband and father.

Returning to our male infant, time after time he will see his mother just before sleeping. She will come when he wakes, wash him and bathe him, dress and undress him, kiss him and cuddle him, tickle him and play boo! She will also take him out and show him off. In those early months and years, his intelligence is only slowly coming to understand the truth of the relationship but meanwhile, his subconscious has been actively but erroneously, grasping the situation from the very beginning though not in an intellectual way, but in an animalistically way. His subconscious recognises the enormous satisfaction of the relationship but takes it for granted assuming it will persist for ever and as it is then, in all respects but especially and significantly, the sexual one.

In the early stage of being sick over his mother, messing or wetting himself and repeatedly calling his mother from her bed at night, will not be viewed as relationship threatening activities. His subconscious however, will eventually realise the importance of keeping the relationship bond strong. The need to strengthen the relationship will be inspired by the slowly-growing perception of a threat to it. The infant begins to recognise a 'rival', a father or brother say, who he begins to notice and also attracts his mother's attention. It is here that jealousy can have its early origins.

Increasingly, the need to compete will give rise to his ambition to make himself more equal and if it is in itself a significant reaction, the male may become, among other possibilities, a workaholic in later life. Should such a man become wealthy despite this, no amount of wealth will be sufficient to satisfy the ambition's need, for a million pounds is as far from totally fulfilling that need as a million is from infinity. However, should the infant feel his need to fulfil the closer bonding or security of relationship urge to be thwarted then that infant may simply 'give-up', resulting in underachieving in life. Alternatively, it might show later as depression or he may begin displaying bad behavioural tendencies and become a 'rebel' in some form.

Sooner or later however, his subconscious is going to realise that the relationship, in the sense it had at first been seen by the male infant who had fought to maintain it, even as circumstances changed, will see it as slipping away. It's rather like desperately holding a precious gem in a dream and trying to hang onto it while waking, he has witnessed his mother's relationship with his father. At first, things that were done had caused no noticeable adverse reactions and he enjoyed only love and security, now he is being told to tell mummy when he needs the potty. Then he is increasingly instructed to do things for himself. Discipline has been encountered. Finally, his self-perception of his importance in that relationship receives the blow of not even being essentially needed at home, for he has his first day at school.

In these views I have concentrated on the negative reaction to events - the positive aspects hardly call for healing techniques, and this series of books is concerned more with the 'what if' and how to bring about beneficial change from the effects of negative experiences. However, it must be stressed that any of these early experiences can have, as normally they will, beneficial effects too. As an example, the child appears to, and genuinely does take a pride in self-achievement and is proud to display his new found independence. At an early age for instance, the child may insist on feeding himself and such compelling urges arise from wanting to be more equal by copying his superiors or competitors. This self-pride in achieving will stand him in good stead as he is egged on, by the positive applause and encouragement his actions brings. The early infantile and juvenile programming, which results from those experiences, will last forever and show themselves in a multitude of ways. The subconscious at birth, like that clean sheet of paper has been much coloured in, and not all attractively so by the age of five or six. Throughout the male's life, he will have a subconscious desire to return to the comfort and security of the loving and happiness experiences of his babyhood, sometimes taking the negative view, with disastrous results with the subconscious perception of failing to be able to do so. In such a case, it may reflect itself either medically or psychologically. By now you may well realise, why so much emphasis is given here to these complexes, for although sexual in their fundamental foundation they also encompass much of what we become.

As illustrations of these early experiences having a significant reaction of a negative nature later in life, I quote the two following cases.

Taking Mother Back Home

The first case was of a very upset travelling salesman who came to me when he met a customer of his - a previous client. He was in his mid-forties and until a month or so before, had been perfectly happy and fit. As the subsequent analysis continued, the case unfurled and the following picture emerged. He was an only child and had a contented life, being brought up in a seaside town. He married and eventually moved many miles away to take up his job which he enjoyed ever since. When his father died, he persuaded his mother to move near to him which she did.

Everything continued smoothly in his life, until one day during a summer, when he found he had only two calls to make and both were back in his old home town. Since they took place on the Friday, he hit upon the idea of taking his mother with him, to stay the weekend looking up old friends. His mother had enthusiastically agreed but without his realising it, a mental 'time bomb' had begun to tick. He suffered a restless night on the Thursday, but didn't know why. The following morning he mentioned to his mother that he felt a 'bit out of sorts', blaming his poor night's sleep.

However, as the journey proceeded he began to feel worse, until he announced to his anxious mother, that he would seek medical help in the next town they came to. Suddenly, he had caused the car to brake heavily, he jumped out and threw himself onto the grass verge, now unable to move. His mother attempted to assist him but found she could do nothing. She stopped a passing car and asked the driver to call an ambulance. Meanwhile, my client reported he had drifted in and out of unconsciousness and knew he was dying. The ambulance arrived and he was rushed to hospital. Over several days and with many checks, nothing was found to be wrong with him and he eventually returned home.

He consulted his doctor who suggested he should resign from his job because it must have been the cause of his stress, and apply to work in the company's office as a precaution against any further such experiences. This he was most reluctant to do, even though he still felt far from normal.

It was at this point that he came to visit me. What I suspect had taken place can never be demonstrated as fact, except in the light of repeated experiences. Knowing that he was to take his mother and have her all to himself on a journey back to his roots, with him having matured to his mother's equal, lead to a connection of subconscious thoughts and memories. Impressing his mother would be the realisation of what he had dreamt of as a boy, being grown up and one day driving his mother in a car-like the ones that came to the seaside. He would be big and important! These thoughts were triggered by his Oedipus complex which had in itself given rise to the objective. Now that objective was realised but clashed with reality and the subconscious programming that had occurred since the creation of the earlier ambition. As a result, the two programmes were to fight an unresolvable battle until that is, he came nearer to an unacceptable point of choice, where his only recourse from the mounting pressure for a subconscious decision, was to collapse and thereby avoid it.

Whether my theorising is accurate or not, the salesman not only fully recovered and sent me several referrals, but accepted promotion to become the company's sales manager and travelled even more widely. Years later I heard that he had set up his own company and was doing very well.

'Ha-Ha Got You!'

In the second case, a male client reported that his teenage son had become increasingly hostile to him over recent years, and he was concerned because this hostility had now become violent. The son agreed to analysis, which was to prove highly successful. The father who was much of the 'family man' type had nevertheless lost his first wife and two children through divorce. He had then met a young widow, who had an eighteen-month-old baby boy. The man was delighted with the prospect of an instant family and the romance blossomed. The widow lived with her mother and the only other two people, who put in frequent appearances, were an aunt and a great aunt of the boy.

The man began giving much playful attention to the boy. The novelty of the man's presence and the subsequent pleasure of the repeated experiences, greatly excited the boy who would eagerly enquire of his mother: "Man come?" "Man come?" A very close bond continued, with the young child to be adopted by the man following the marriage. However, the relationship between the man and boy was to settle down to a normal happy one, with the original intensity of the father's attention gradually reducing as the boy aged.

Subconsciously the boy grew increasingly annoyed with the perceived loss when comparing the reality of his emerging adulthood with the delights of his babyhood. The subconscious frustration had mounted, ultimately bringing his father to his predicament. In short, the subconscious of the teenager still had a longing to be picked up, swung in the air, to be kissed and hugged, played with, tickled and tricked, loved and encouraged - all as if a baby.

The relationship between the two, I'm happy to report, is an excellent one today. A further interesting aspect of the case was that the teenager, then nineteen, had increasingly been suffering a painful right knee. His doctor said it was caused by 'wear and tear', and that nothing could be done, although the son was far from the physically active type. During analysis, it transpired that the last physical demonstrations of the early affection was the sudden grasping of the boys right knee by the father, while saying loudly "Ha-Ha, got you!"

On the occasions they drove alone in the car together. Somehow this action became a representation of those earlier experiences which gave rise to much pleasure for both. The subsequent perceived loss was focused onto this act, the last demonstrated affection of its kind. The negative effect of the loss was felt by the boy's subconscious and reflected back to his knee, resulting in a state that had made walking for more than a few hundred yards too painful to endure.

Following analysis the knee pain was also to go and the son is now an active squash player- and a good one at that! Whilst this case is not of the Oedipus origin, it has nevertheless been included to illustrate the powerful effects of early relationships. By adding the enormously powerful sexual factor - had it been a mother figure that arrived on the scene, meeting a widowed father, living with other male family members, then the same reaction from her would have triggered the Oedipus Complex. Had the mother then withdrawn her physically expressed actions in the same way as the man, then in addition to any other reactions that may have resulted there could have arisen misogynistic or sodimistic tendencies, which are in themselves, the outcome of the Oedipus Complex in some cases anyway.

I Can't Move House

As a further illustration of the Oedipus Complex at work, the case of a man orphaned as a baby comes to mind, let's call him Harry. While growing up he developed the same aspirations as his fellows that one day, as happened from time to time with others, a couple would come down the long orphanage drive and he would be summoned to the office and introduced to them. This would be the forerunner of visits to the couple's home, with the hopeful result of eventual adoption.

Gone would be the dormitory and being just one of a number in its place would be caring parents, a room of his own and a family life like most boys and girls enjoy. Time after time he saw others realise their ambition. He envied the lucky ones who boasted of their experiences as they became established on their road to a 'natural' home life. Eagerly, Harry waited to participate in this adventure as well though often fearing he may not, since such a happy fate had eluded others, whom he saw approaching their teens and still resident. One day to his considerable delight, he was summoned to the office, only moments before having seen just such a couple approach. He was introduced to the couple and was much taken by them. The hoped for outings took place until the even more hoped for question was posed - would he like them to be his new mummy and daddy? The excitement experienced as the outings continued, while final arrangements were made, was enormous and culminated in his leaving the orphanage with his small parcel of personal possessions. He recalled looking back and waving to the faces he knew would be watching and envying him as he strode excitedly, and for the last time, up that long drive - just as he had watched others do so in the past.

Harry was not to know that his subconscious had bonded him to a nurse who had played a major role in caring for him at the orphanage. Soon after his settling in his new home, he began to become ever more restless and seemed anxious. The couple's doctor suggested that this was to be expected in such changed circumstances and that he would soon settle down, make new friends and acclimatise.

But Harry got worse. One day, by now seven years old, he suddenly and impulsively stabbed himself in the testicles with scissors. Although he survived the incident medically well enough, his new parents were seriously concerned with what was wrong, and wondered if they made an awful mistake. Fortunately, Harry finally began to settle down, much to the relief of all. Life continued normally until the time came for him, as was usual in those days, to be called up for his compulsory eighteen months national service in the armed forces.

Soon after joining up, he experienced a growing anxiety. To his subconscious, he had not just left home but was reminded of the earlier situation when he had left his nurse at the orphanage. He was again compelled to stab himself in the testicles, this time even more seriously. Shortly after he was medically discharged and returned home, once again becoming his normal self. Eventually he was to meet and marry an attractive young lady. When they left to

43

live in their first home - having started their marriage living with his parents, he was once again to attack himself as previously, again medically surviving the experience. There was one further similar repetition when Harry and his wife subsequently moved home once more. The undoubted conclusion, to one and all, was that Harry had a bizarre psychological reaction to moving and the remedy suggested by his psychiatrist, and readily accepted by Harry, was never to move again.

Over the following years Harry did well and despite his previous self-inflicted injuries, managed to become a father of two children. Life was good, Harry was promoted then promoted further. With promotion Harry found himself too distant from where he ought to be living for his job, and he tired of the excessive travelling each day. He was forced to consider moving. Warily, the concept of a potential move was approached.

All seemed all right until an actual meeting took place with the estate agent to discuss buying a new home. Within hours, he was aware of the old familiar feelings of agitation and immediately telephoned the estate agent to cancel the project. It was soon after, by way of a last resort, as it often is, that Harry consulted me. Following a successful analysis, he was eventually able to move home with none of his previous experiences. One rather sad note came to the surface however, on looking back he realised that the memories of the nurse, back in the orphanage, had frequently intruded into his thoughts, even over all the years since he last saw her. Now he realised why, and was to cry as he told me that he had only learnt by chance, that she had died the year before.

The reader may feel that some of the cases reported are barely believable and yet they are true, only distorted enough to protect and guard against any possibility of the clients being identified. However, the cases are examples of the consequences of a fundamental condition, that to a greater or lesser extent, mostly rests in all of us. The question is not if we are the subject of the complex but to what extent we are.

Complications arising from the Complexes

If the subconscious has too fixed an impression of the mother or mother figure as a partner, then he may never marry as no woman would be able to meet his exacting requirements. He may marry but unfulfillingly so. His marriage may end in failure or he may become a womaniser, that is without realising it, he may remain constantly searching for a satisfaction of the subconscious need, that can never actually be achieved. In short, the complex can easily be the basis of what is commonly known as relationship difficulties. The male could become impotent because the sexual act may be thought of, by the subconscious, as an adulterous act, his mother, to his subconscious being the real partner.

Although, as illustrated in Book Three of this series of books, impotency can have other origins. For similar reasons, the inability or difficulty to climax may result. Premature ejaculation may occur with a bizarre 'quick before its too late' reaction, perhaps reflecting a sense of missed opportunities in early life. Sometimes a male will be sexually physically aggressive, stemming from a revengeful reaction to being aroused by the female which could result from his subconsciously being reminded of the sexual power his mother once had over him. Shyness, in both male and female, particularly when dealing with the opposite sex, mostly has its origins in the 'guilty' thoughts of the subconscious and conscious minds in earlier times.

The evidence of the Oedipus Complex may never show itself, or be greatly delayed in doing so and only come to the surface following some triggering event. Alternatively the aggravation caused by it can have profound medical or physiological effects as well as psychological. Where the effect is sufficient and is expressed physiologically, the consequences can range from the insignificant and go through a comprehensive list of medical symptoms which may have, at its other end of the scale, death as a result, say by heart attack in an otherwise normally healthy person. For instance, the termination of the means of fulfilling an ambition, say by retirement or by once again coming upon the never resolved complex suddenly in sleep, may produce that result from the shock that it creates. Where the subconscious effect exists in any significant degree, the victim will be carrying a mental 'load' or suffer a de-harmonising mind state. Consequently, a sufficiently subsequent emotive experience will be an additional load or an additional de-harmonising event, and may combine to become unendurable and in some way producing a symptom - the combination possibly producing what is commonly referred to as a nervous breakdown for example, or in the physiological sense cause a person to look worried. Such victims are rarely aware of the basic mental load they carry and so never make any connection.

In my practice I have come across many psychologically and physiological conditions produced in this way. Inevitably it comes as a surprise for the client to discover a connection between their malady and the repressed experience of their complex.

Whilst the Oedipus Complex can result in a seemingly limitless list of negative conditions, I feel compelled to mention a few more of the many benefits among which are the sense of competition generally such as in sports, ambition, determination and personal achievement, all beneficial to society at large and commonly having their origins in the complexes. Some people claim they know the time and cause of their becoming, say, determined. I suggest that it was some subsequent event or circumstance triggering into action, that otherwise dormant or latent programme. Without doubt, the strongest beneficial reaction is the wish to marry and thereby come as close as possible to secure the nearest version of that early relationship. In marriage a man may subconsciously look for a partner who will remind him of his mother in some way as if some distant echo of her, although most men would consciously deny it vigorously. The male victim of the complex, given the right partner, particularly in oral characters, can produce the most loyal and dedicated of husbands. In marriage society benefits from the security of the children having the protection, teaching, encouragement and support which will lead them into responsible adulthood where they in their turn, will duplicate the principle and consequently perpetuate and preserve the species.

The Electra Complex

Named after Electra's devotions to Agamemnon in the Greek legend, the Electra Complex is similar to that of the male infants Oedipus Complex but normally the father is selected. However, the chosen male partner may easily be another and be the grandfather, brother, uncle or other male acquaintance. The male partner will be the one providing the greatest fascination, and the female infant can, as with the male infant, be regarded as being infatuated. In both, this infatuation will normally be redirected to another in adulthood with the desire for a partner of the opposite sex. However, the echoes of the earlier Electra Complex encounter, in some ways, will remain forever and with as many possible consequences as the male may encounter from his Oedipus Complex. The infatuation, subconsciously, may be reflected back, respectively by the infants mother or selected male, and in this too, there may be a residual effect in the parent.

Much of what can be said of the male Oedipus Complex,

can also be said of the female Electra Complex version. However and inevitably there are major differences in the effects produced, and this is because of the fundamental differences in the mental and physiological make-up of the two sexes and of course, during its construction, a powerful but same sex relationship exists between mother and daughter. Initially a significant male figure may be absent or the one who is present, may not inspire the depth of emotion to trigger the Electra Complex response.

Under these last two circumstances the female will either 'await' the arrival of a suitable male, or grow up with little or no attraction to men. She may become bisexual or lesbian or even anti-male. Such reactions of course, can also result from a genuinely stimulated Electra Complex but be the distorted results of it. Such reactions may be further compounded, should the growing female infant come to realise with her developing intelligence, that the selected male figure is unacceptable or even repulsive in some way, or that in maturity no male, either meets her expectations or excites her by comparison. More commonly than the absence of the mother of the boy, the father may have far less contact, be absent or simply over involved with his work.

When the female infant feels rejected or ignored by her father, she may lose herself-confidence, adopt an attitude of self-dislike or many other symptoms could appear. To attract her father's attention, the little girl will want to be seen as pretty, clever and talented. In the switch of her affection from her mother to her father, a sense of betrayal may be induced, giving rise to the repeating dreams of pursuer or threats that the male experiences.

The early experiences are more complex in the female compared to the male perhaps because of this, and coupled with her natural tendencies to be more emotionally aware, there may be some clue as to why the female is more vulnerable to neurotic conditions and symptoms than is the male. Initially all the daughter's love is reflected back to her mother. The sexual aspect, given they are of the same sex, will normally be non existent. Where the sexual aspect is included, it too may give rise to bisexuality or lesbianistic tendencies later in life, particularly when it occurs in the absence of a suitable male attraction.

A similar result can be caused by an over indulgent mother who continues her intensive attentions over a protracted period of time. In this latter case, the maturing female may fall between two stones, not knowing in which direction to proceed, as if suffering from some inner loss of purposefulness. As a result she may simply find marriage lacking in satisfaction or appeal, though remaining basically heterosexual.

Much more often however the female infant, following the subconscious realisation that her infatuation with the selected male partner cannot remain a reality, will want to return to the satisfying security of the earlier experience which existed prior to her mental adventure. She returns with a subconscious sense of shame or guilt and may be inclined, subconsciously, to try to make up for her competition for mother's husband, by making efforts to befriend her - this is a much rarer reaction of the male to his father. Such befriending by the daughter can be taken to enormous lengths. In some cases where, like the male not being satisfied will his million pounds, she may never feel that she has achieved an acceptable level of friendship to meet her needs.

Where the daughter's friendship is rejected or not returned to the degree to which it is offered, enormous consequences of anxiety can follow. In some cases, this need can sometimes express itself by the daughter acquiring a female friend, with a great bond of friendship being pursued. Alternatively, this powerful need for a bond with another female, may take the form of an excellent and fulfilling relationship with the mother of her husband. This friendship or bonding by the daughter can have enormous benefits in both child rearing and looking after elderly mothers.

Overweight in women will often have its origins in the Electra Complex, being the self-compensating reaction to it. In the male Oedipus Complex we looked at impotency as an effect, in just the same way in the female, frigidity or the inability to orgasm may result and not necessarily because of the incompetence of the male partner. So too, in a similar way that the male may 'chase' women, the female may 'go for anything in trousers'.

Other adverse effects can also occur, for example, where otherwise everything is as it should be, the inability to conceive may result, be delayed or even miscarriages take place. For conception itself may be considered as adulterous to her subconscious mind. As an alternative, a difficult pregnancy or childbirth may have its origins in the complex. Everything else may go smoothly in the pregnancy and childbirth stages, but the mother may then find she cannot love the child that is born to her because to her subconscious, it is not her father's offspring. Although more commonly, this lack of a natural ability to love her offspring arises because the mother herself was unloved as a child, and she finds it difficult to pass on that which she never had herself.

It is the same perceived infidelity or adulterous subconscious perception which could be the foundation of some vaginal and breast cancers. If the boy and his 'knee' example quoted earlier is recalled, the possibility must at least exist that such conditions and perhaps many others, especially gynaecological ones, may have their origins in the Electra Complex, particularly when one considers the bodily locations of initial sexual encounters, such theorising cannot be automatically excluded from serious consideration.

It is also possible that the subconscious could consider initial sexual encounters as guilt-laden or adulterous acts, and mentally identify them in those locations, especially since the female takes relationships more seriously. As a further possibility, and as if of some perverse contortion of her natural sense of relationship loyalty, her subconscious might be tempted to destroy her marriage, remaining fixed on her early infatuation and subconsciously seeing it threatened, challenged or disloyally misplaced by a mature second relationship.

For the subconscious can and does in some cases, find ways of destroying that secondary relationship. In this case the relationship is considered 'adulterous' and has to be terminated. When this happens either her subconscious reacts adversely to end it or causes the male to react in some way to achieve that same objective. The following three cases are quoted to illustrate some of the complications the Electra Complex can produce.

Holding Hands Under the Table

An intelligent, attractive and sophisticated lady reported to me that she was the victim of a totally mysterious condition, one which defied all her intellect and ran totally contrary to all her normal sense of behaviour. Encouraged to go on, she explained that at about monthly intervals she would have an irresistible urge - which she always eventually succumbed to, to ring her brother and arrange to meet him. They would then meet in a quiet back room of the country pub, which they had selected for such occasions being many miles away it had the advantage that they wouldn't be known by anyone. "We go in, my brother buys our drinks and soon afterwards we hold hands under the table and quietly weep. After another drink we'll take the long journey home. Sometimes, while attempting to resist the temptation to ring him, my brother will ring me to arrange to meet. Either way, it comes to the same thing and heavens above, there's no sexual factor".

During analysis, both the Electra and Oedipus Complexes were explained, with her being treated for the Electra version. She immediately realised what had been going on, and that during their happy childhood they had developed the two complexes for each other. She also realised that her brother's first marriage was broken up by it and that his second marriage, together with her marriage, was being subconsciously broken up too. Subsequently I treated the brother and each reported a harmonising of their marriages and an end of the need of their secret meetings.

'Why do I put up with this Crap?'

In the cases reported, I often refer to the clients as intelligent, attractive or achievers, such references are deliberate. They serve the point of emphasising, firstly that intelligence has little beneficial effect in such matters and secondly, that the complexes spare no particular types, as this next case underlines. A vivacious, intelligent and talented lady from the entertainment world consulted me and reported how frequently her work took her on overseas tours, where she would be admired and applauded and her social company much sought after.

Although happily married, she was greatly upset by an irresistible urge that occurred on completing each tour, to telephone her father before her husband. She would tell him how it had gone and that she was returning to Britain and looked forward to seeing him again. She was upset because on each such occasion her father would respond to her call enthusiastically, but sooner or later, he would descend into great abusiveness of her. He would begin by accusing her of having been 'off whoring' and go on in this vein until almost without exception, the lady would be forced to bang the phone down on him. Despite all this, on her return, she would find herself urged to visit her father as soon as possible, with the inevitable result of the visit becoming a re-run of the telephone experience. With tears running down her face, she shouted: "I'm held in such high esteem, I'm at the peak of my career - why do I put up with this crap?"

By now the reader requires little further explanation of course. Once again I am happy to report that her relationship is on a far better level as a result of her treatment. An additional point of interest in this case, was that with the knowledge she gained in the sessions, she found an explanation of a situation which had puzzled her for years. "Why was it", she often wondered, "the female dancers with whom she frequently worked, were so 'man mad' after their performances?" - well, the desire to be attractive to satisfy their Electra Complex needs, was being fulfilled by their act of dancing and being applauded.

The resultant reaction would be the need for male companionship, for the females would then be at least subconsciously, extensively aroused. My lady client realised with her open-minded intelligence, what was going on. "My God", she said "now I realise, I can see it all, this is going on all around me!"

'He Can't Get an Erection'

One afternoon, a wealthy couple came to consult me and sat side by side in front of my desk. They had given no previous indication for their wishing to see me. In a matter of fact way they explained that they were father and daughter and were having an affair, which had finally resulted in the wife leaving, and so they decided to live unrestrictedly as man and wife. "But", interjected the daughter "now we have what we want, he (pointing accusingly at her father) can't get an erection!" It was this impotency they wanted 'sorting out'. I did not see myself in a position to judge or advise them in anyway, but I saw an enormous potential hazard in my resolving his impotency problem. Since it would be unlikely I would also be invited to treat the daughter, I foresaw the 'risk' of unlocking her father from the relationship in the course of releasing him from the ramifications of the complexes, that would be necessary to restore his potency. What was going on in him, was either that his subconscious was responding to the repulsion of the relationship, or his heightened emotional state had reactivated his Oedipus Complex relationship with his own mother.

Whichever is the basic reason for his impotency, a successful treatment was most likely to result in breaking his relationship with his daughter in its then form, while leaving his daughter still clinging to it in its former state. Fortunately, while crossing my fingers that I might find a solution to the dilemma, I was released by the client telephoning and leaving a message on my answer phone cancelling his next appointment. I have never heard from them since.

Parental Reactions to the Complexes

Another aspect of the two complexes that also calls for open mindedness and insight, is the possibility of the reactions from the infant's selected partner. The infant will not only experience the infatuation, but will also subconsciously transmit the message back of being infatuated. Many possible consequences of such transmissions can occur. Among these are that the transmissions will be subconsciously received, understood and accepted by the receiver, who may then be triggered to respond by transmitting back that the feelings are mutual. But the feelings in the selected partner, will be vastly less intense than those of the infant.

However, that intensity will be likely to develop as the infant grows and matures. Eventually, in some ironic twist, the intensity could even become greater in the selected partner than in the now mature but former infant. However, both are normally to remain locked into one another, almost irrespective of subsequent events and for the remainder of the life of each. In the Oedipus Complex the mother may develop the view that no woman is good enough for her son, and become possessive of him, with the same view being taken by the father of the daughter, in the Electra Complex version.

The maturing and developing female will seek to experiment with clothes and make-up, to appear more attractive, the father's subconscious might then respond by desiring a fulfilment of the mutual bond in a sexual way, i.e., the father now finds himself subconsciously sexually drawn to his daughter, and mostly without realising it consciously. Such a reaction may result in profound inner conflict in the father, with him being totally unaware of what's happening or why he feels as he does. Sometimes the reaction results in a complicated conflict. The father may then express his displeasure in the way the daughter dresses, presents herself, develops her social life and to him, the horror that his daughter is beginning to have boy friends. The father however, may quickly adjust, by reverting to pride in her.

Alternatively, the situation may develop where the daughter can do no right, constant rows, disputes, arguments and fault-finding can occur, forcing the daughter to seek an escape by leaving home, with her urge to do so further heightened perhaps, by the mother's subconscious jealousy factor stemming from earlier years, when she witnessed the Electra Complex being mutually laid down between father and daughter. The mother may also resent the presence of the developing and prettier younger woman with all the freedom she has.

55

Each are victims, none the villain. In another aspect, the partner of the one selected, being of the same sex as the infant, will become aware of the initial transmissions taking place between the two and react, most likely with subconscious jealousy. The extent of the feelings and the rows which follow, might develop to the degree that the marriage might even break down. Should this occur, particularly with the young male offspring, a subsequent suitor may be in for a very difficult time indeed.

In the Oedipus Complex the father may respond to his jealousy in a variety of ways; he may become impatient and distressed by his male offspring; or develop an open resentment. The child may respond to what he now sees as his rival's hostility, by becoming rebellious, which may spill over from the father to son conflict and into society at large in some way, perhaps commencing with minor infringements of school rules.

He may even progress to vandalism or stealing from shops but always driven on by the once started, but never resolved Oedipus Complex-based mind state, although his activities may change. Given more interesting options, such as the entry into his life of a sufficiently appealing girlfriend or some occupational opportunity giving sufficient job satisfaction, he may simply grow out of his ways, or perhaps be spurred on to do so when ultimately, he may find himself threatened by imprisonment.

Of course, the developing child will also respond very significantly in line with his character type. The reactions of the Orals may be of depression, withdrawal, under-achieving and lacking motivation and enthusiasm. The Anal will tend to be more vocal, deliberately provocative - particularly as he enters his teens and he may become violent or the school bully. With the Anal, the situation will be likely to deteriorate should the mother, responding to the Oedipus-based bond, be seen to openly take the son's side. The Genital may react with martyrdom, irresponsibility, criminality, seeking to direct the reactions onto someone or something else, like illness or inventing some situation. Reactions are further complicated and compounded by the left/right brain balances of those involved together with their degrees of intelligence. The Anals and Genitals may even resort to murdering a parent or parents, especially if some financial or other gain is an added incentive. Probably half of the male prisoners would be found to have the negative driving force of the Oedipus Complex as the basic condition leading to their imprisonment.

Where the jealousy is between mother and daughter, similar reactions to those of the father and son relationship may evolve. Mothers in this situation can be more outspoken and effective in what they may say. The mother may extend her jealousy into perceiving her daughter as a hussy and begin accusing her of this or that. Eventually, in some cases, the daughter can respond by becoming pregnant, serving the joint purpose of responding to her mother's accusations by defiantly turning them into truths, and enabling the daughter to leave home and gain freedom.

In Conclusion

At the beginning of this chapter, the difficulty of writing about the subject was referred to, with part of that difficulty coming from the sheer enormity of the task and reducing such a vast subject to a single chapter. Despite this, it is to be hoped that some indication of the huge value of incorporating the complexes in treatment, as given in session six of the analysis, has been justified.

Some may still think much of this is highly-blown theory, but that carries with it the risk of missing a vital part of the human puzzle, in a similar way to a jigsaw puzzle, not every part fits every space but that doesn't mean the part held fits no space at all. All of the theory parts need to be available just in case any do fit you or your client. If the theory does fit, and you have previously rejected it, the outcome of the analysis will be incomplete. Accept these concepts and find they do not fit or are irrelevant, and nothing will be lost. They are not put forward to the client as some input to a subject's mind, no more than that puzzle piece, of the wrong shape, allows you to put that piece in place.

Don't expect intelligent modern reactions from a non-intellectual mind, that is mainly still running on a programme laid down in the very first years of life. A further point which must be stressed and emphasised, is that if you are one of those females unlucky enough to have a father you grew up to detest, it does not mean you can have no Electra Complex link with him. The Electra Complex is laid down before the intellectual mind is sufficiently mature enough to evaluate him. Besides, there could just as easily have been another male.

As the reader also will - should he help others - I come across cases where the unfortunate female is in the awful situation of both being drawn to the father and also feeling a repulsion of him. Since the feeling of being drawn to him comes from the highly effective subconscious and the rejection from the conscious the resolution, in one way or the other, will be difficult for her. You may have heard of an unhappy daughter feeling trapped at home, taking care of an ungrateful father, as an example. The effects of each complex may only come into effect when some conflicting experience takes place, marriage, divorce, leaving home, having a child, losing a parent or the break-up of a relationship.

However, there is an additional major factor that sets the neurosis resulting from the complexes apart from the neurotic conditions otherwise encountered. This additional factor is that they are generated in the subconscious and by the subconscious with intellectual assessment having played little initial part. The child may react in a jealous way to a brother or sister say, but that will be the response to the earlier programming, not the cause of the reduced value of the relationship, even if it is to add to the intensity of the programme, so that the reactions become more apparent.

The uniqueness of the two complexes rests in their having been constructed in the subconscious, and not having entered the mind via an emotional and intellectually experienced situation. Because of this, during analysis the resolving of the complexes cannot be experienced in the conscious mind and are therefore not (abreacted) Consequently the client will have no way of knowing if the complex is relevant to them at the time of release or even of the extent to which it is! This is not to prevent the benefits which follow but sometimes however, a person will have good reasons for suspecting they may be the victim of the relevant complex.

During analysis, any emotive response will be the release of emotions associated with their complex, rather than of the complex itself, i.e., from any subsequent complex initiated emotional experiences. Because of the lack of any apparent reaction to the complex release, it is very useful to support the release in a second but different way. Both the release and the additional release support methods are given in the details of analysis.

When the seemingly limitless varieties of expressions and symptoms the complexes can create, is added to the extent of their potential effects, I feel justified in my claim that they are the greatest single source of human misery in the world, with all their potential for physiological and psychological damage, even travelling thousands of miles, to attend the single hour's session needed to release them, would be worth all the cost and effort. Imagine a country, or eventually the world where their release became standard preventative medicine? What then the quality of life for society as a whole?

59

Chapter Three

Dealing Directly with the Subconscious

Using the concept of the mind running the body, some amazingly useful and very impressive techniques can be employed, to contact the subconscious directly. These techniques by-pass the intellectual conscious mind and thereby help eliminate the risk of the client's conscious interference. The techniques can be used to question the subconscious or to discuss and verify given issues that might otherwise be difficult or even impossible to resolve in other ways often producing instead, astounding results.

To understand the principles involved, we need to remind ourselves again of the personality and thought mechanisms of the subconscious which may have different thoughts, values, priorities, reactions, understandings, needs and principles to the conscious mind. We also need to remind ourselves that the subconscious can have a fundamentally different personality to the conscious mind although more normally the subconscious will reflect the personality of the conscious and may in some respects, be more emphatic on some issues or even hold totally opposing views. For instance, the person may consciously wish to stop smoking while the subconscious wishes to continue. The conscious may wish to continue to live but the subconscious not to. In some extreme cases the subconscious may even dislike the conscious mind and the person he has become. The conscious mind may be inspired to study, gain promotion, earn more money or follow a particular occupation, while the subconscious feels over-taxed with the aggravation of so doing. In relationships too, the subconscious may disagree with the selection of a partner by the conscious. The subconscious may disagree with the desire of the conscious mind to fulfil sexual intentions resulting for example, in impotency. The subconscious may be concerned with some matter the conscious is not, thus producing a symptom or condition representing its worry and concern. The point in all this is simple, it should never be assumed that the subconscious is simply a mirror image of the conscious, because it is not. The reason for stressing and repeating this concept, is because it is essential for the therapists to be consciously aware of it at all times. The revelation of this difference often comes as a complete surprise to the client. The hypnotherapist using the direct contact techniques will constantly come across examples of this difference during therapy.

In both of the first methods of contacting the subconscious directly, there is a restriction of the information retrievable, in that only a 'yes' or 'no' reply is available, resulting in a need to put questions in a simple form that clearly do call for such a response. Furthermore, several such questions may be needed in order to retrieve the information required. This potentially protracted enquiry method therefore requires the therapist to keep a good mental track of the progress, especially since the subconscious is reluctant to repeat itself by answering the same basic question twice. At a conscious level you might ask someone to do something with him agreeing to do so. You may then check with him that he doesn't mind, and be reassured by him that he doesn't. Following this, you might go on to say you would understand if he did object with him responding by reassuring you once again, that he does not. Should such a sequence of asking and checking be attempted with the subconscious only the first question would elicit a response with the checking questions being ignored. That is unless some sound logical reason could be given for a further similar response. Notwithstanding these points enormously helpful information can be obtained where the subconscious co-operates, as mostly it does in response to being requested to do so.

The Hand-Holding Technique
The 'Neurological Idio Motor Response

Technically, this is a version of an idio motor response, or I.M.R. In this a third person is to hold the client's right hand, because the client is more likely to be right-handed and therefore likely to be more responsive with it, although the left hand may also be used. The hand is held in a 'sandwich' fashion by the third person with both palms turned towards the clients hand. When the client and assistant are both in a comfortable position, with the client having his eyes closed, the subconscious is requested to respond in the following way.

Therapist: "Subconscious, in a moment I am going to ask you some important questions for (*client's name*) benefit". "Here is how I want you to respond". "If your answer to a question is 'yes' then I want you to cause a nerve in (*client's name*) right hand to jump, twitch or react in a clear positive and unmistakable way". "If, however, your answer is 'no' then I want you to do nothing". "Subconscious, you make the 'yes' signal as clear as the effect that we all experience from time to time, when a nerve jumps or twitches on the inside of the knee". "Subconscious, I want you to select the nerve now that you intend to use and cause just such a reaction to say 'yes' to show that you have".

Note: Some persuasion may be required if the response is not initially received. Sometimes it is necessary for the third person to change the position of their hands to cover some other area of the client's hand. The signal may for instance, be occurring in the tip of one finger rather than the more usual response occurring in the client's palm or back of his hand.

Where difficulties continue to be experienced, the client should be asked if he can feel the response and if so, where it is located. Sometimes the response will be in his arm and not reach the hand, being felt only there. About half of all clients will be able to detect the signals themselves, the other half remaining unaware of them. Signal strength will vary with enthusiasm, and this will be especially noticeable the nearer the therapist comes to the point of some subconscious interest or concern. In some cases, the subconscious can become so enthusiastic that it causes the reaction to be almost continuous. In this reaction, the subconscious is responding with a 'yes, yes, yes, yes' type of response.

Sadly, such enthusiasm is not entirely helpful for in these cases, the subconscious may not respond with the appropriate 'nos', remaining only concerned with the 'yes, yes, yes, yes', - 'you've got it', 'that's it', or 'I do want to' reactions. The third party, so as not to distract the client's subconscious, is to indicate the replies received from the hand by nodding or shaking their head. Consequently, the therapist is to observe both of them, and can best do so by sitting on the client's left so that both the client and the assistant are in the therapist's natural line of sight. The assistant may vocalise the response in cases where the client cannot feel the reactions.

One slightly amusing occurrence is when the client, consciously wishing to co-operate, physically moves part of his hand to indicate a 'yes' answer. Not only is such a reaction easily detectable by the assistant, but it will often be at variance with the actual answer given by the subconscious. Where this happens, the subconscious response should be taken as the true answer. This rarely-known of technique is reliable, because it completely eliminates the possibility of any conscious interference being undetected by the assistant.

Note too that consciously, the client can neither cause such a spontaneous reaction nor prevent it. (Try doing so with that nerve reaction in the inside of the knee, should you seek confirmation).

There are two further substantial advantages of the technique. Not only can it be used equally effectively without hypnosis being induced - although the client should have his eyes closed to aid concentration, but also a third person participating as the intermediator gives the client a far greater confidence in the procedure, particularly so where the third person is an acquaintance of the client and especially if either are sceptical.

A disadvantage of the method is that it does normally require three people to use it. One further point of consideration is that the subconscious may be disinclined to co-operate with the selected assistant, especially in the case where the assistant is a relative and because of this, having a partner in a hypnotherapy practice is a major advantage. It is also an advantage to have a female assistant as she is more likely to have sensitive hands. Where initial reluctance is encountered, a little patience and effort can still produce good results - in all but exceptional instances. In some cases, the 'yes' signals may suddenly cease and when they do it can indicate that the subconscious has withdrawn from further communication - rather like he might put a phone down on a caller he no longer wishes to speak to.

The first two sequences to follow have been deliberately complicated in order to illustrate the technique itself and the method of overcoming a reluctance to respond whereas in the vast majority of cases it is a remarkably straightforward technique. In the way explained earlier, the 'yes' signal has been requested but has failed to materialise. The therapist continues:

Therapist: "Subconscious, the signal was not detected, please send the signal that would mean 'yes' once again".

Note: If there is no response the third person is invited to move his hand-holding position.

Therapist: "Subconscious please send that 'yes' signal now". (no response) "Subconscious, I know that you are busy and normally don't repeat yourself but this issue is so important that I ask you to make an exception. If you have sent that signal and it has been missed, I would rather run the risk of offending you by asking you to repeat your signal than I would run the risk of letting (*client's name*) down. Please send that signal again". (no response)

Note: The subject should be asked if he has felt the signal at this stage and if he has, the assistant is to relocate their hands accordingly if necessary, and the subconscious is then requested to signal 'yes' once again. If such a location is not indicated by the client continue along the following lines.

Therapist: "Subconscious, please make an exception to your apparent reluctance to co-operate by using that 'yes' signal, to respond to my next question. No offence will be taken if you say 'yes'. Subconscious, are you reluctant to co-operate with me through (*assistant's name*)?"

Note: If 'Yes', reassure the subconscious and stressing the importance of helping (*client's name*) and that no embarrassing questions will be asked - a reassurance that will often succeed, where initial requests for co-operation fail, and especially in cases where the assistant is neutral. An alternative or additional question to the last one, and one that often does produce positive results in such situations is:

Therapist: "Subconscious, are you afraid?"

Note: Commonly, in such situations of initial difficulty, the response will be 'Yes', and subsequently encouragement should be given. A method which often succeeds, is one of reassuring the subconscious by explaining what it is concerned with, is just an old memory, and that since (*client's name*) survived the original experience (*client's name*) can easily deal with only the memory of it.

Therapist: "Besides subconscious (*client's name*) intelligent mind will find it nothing like as important as you did. You are not on

65

your own now and perfectly safe in here. Subconscious, when (*client's name*) knows what that memory is, his symptoms will go away restoring peace and harmony. You are then free of it too. Subconscious, please send that 'yes' signal now, to confirm we can proceed".

Note: More often than not the response will be 'Yes' and the outcome will be successful. However, where further efforts continue to produce negative results, either a replacement assistant should be tried where possible, or the attempt eventually be terminated. Actually, as stated previously, the method is normally very easy to use and can be highly productive, especially in sessions seven and eight of analysis. With analysis cases that have otherwise proved difficult, the technique can often prove to be the turning point and lead to success.The technique can also be most useful with a subject who misunderstands his role properly, or has some other obstacle in his way, such as a pronounced inability to detect or visualise information passed to him from his subconscious.

To further illustrate the technique, the following example of the procedure is given. Harry reported that his right arm became so painful, following a road accident, that he could no longer drive. All medical examinations, x-rays and tests indicated nothing was wrong. Physiotherapy had also failed and the analysis had brought no significant benefit either. Halfway through session seven, it was decided to try the hand-holding technique and readily the subconscious responded with the 'Yes' signal, to the request to co-operate.

Therapist: "Subconscious please carry out an inspection of Harry's right arm and say 'yes' when you have".
(A few seconds pause)
Client: "Yes".
Therapist: "Good. Thank you subconscious, is Harry's right arm physically damaged?"
Client: "No".

Note: If the answer had been 'yes', then the mind over matter self-healing technique, described in Book Three of this series would have been called for.

Therapist: "Then subconscious, is Harry's arm condition caused by some Psychological cause".

Client: "Yes".

Therapist: "Thank you subconscious. Subconscious, is that psychological cause specifically due to Harry's car accident?"

Client: "No".

Therapist: "Is it connected with it in some way?"

Client: "Yes".

Therapist: "Then is the condition also the result of an earlier experience?"

Client: "Yes".

Therapist: "Subconscious I'll count to three and click my fingers, and you bring into Harry's mind what that earlier cause is". "One, two, three, click".

Client: Reports nothing remembered.

Therapist: "Subconscious you clearly know what that earlier experience was, so would you actually confirm that you do?"

Client: "Yes".

Therapist: "Good, did you send a memory of that occasion to Harry just now?"

Client: "Yes".

Therapist: "Harry then what did you see?"

Client: "Nothing".

Therapist: "Subconscious, would you agree to send that memory to Harry again?"

Client: "Yes".

Therapist: "One, two, three ,click". (Harry becomes visually uncomfortable) "What is it Harry?"

Client: "I remember putting my arm around my younger brother's neck, while I stood behind him and tried to strangle him".

Therapist: "Subconscious do you feel guilty over that incident?"

Client: "Yes".

Therapist: "Would you agree to release that guilty tension, and let Harry be free from it?"

Client: "No".

Therapist: "Subconscious, Harry can easily handle that release, and he would never try to strangle his brother again".

Client reacts: Harry's right eye suddenly releases four tear drops. (pause)

Therapist: "Subconscious, have you released that guilt now?"

Client: "Yes".

Note: Such a spontaneous release can often happen, and in such a release, the right eye will cry. If no release had occurred at this point, further similar negotiations would have followed, and could have continued as follows.

Therapist: "Subconscious, does Harry get any benefit from that guilt?"

Client: "Yes".

Therapist: "Does it protect him?"

Client: "No".

Therapist: "Does it serve another purpose?"

Client: "Yes".

Therapist: "Does it cause him to be punished in some way?"

Client: "Yes".

Note: To the unintelligent subconscious, guilt may beget punishment, and where punishment is decided upon, the logic of the subconscious is that the guilt remaining unresolved, self punishment needs to be continued.

Therapist: "Is that punishment the reason for Harry's arm condition?"

Client: "No".

Therapist: "Is it part of the reason for the condition?"

Client:	"Yes".
Therapist:	"Good. Subconscious, Harry desperately needs his arm restoring to good health, and I call upon you to release him from his punishment, so will you now agree to release him?"
Client:	"No".
Therapist:	"Subconscious would you agree that if Harry's guilt was released, there would no longer be any reason for punishment?"
Client:	"Yes".
Therapist:	"Subconscious, every punishment, even for serious crimes, must come to an end at some time, that is so isn't it?"
Client:	"Yes".
Therapist:	"This punishment has gone on too long and it is too severe, and needs to be terminated, so that Harry can get on with his life, do you agree with that?"
Client:	"Yes".
Therapist:	"Then will you now release Harry?"

Client reacts: Initially with a short hesitation, (any hesitation is detectable, by the nerve neither expressing 'yes' or 'no'. Rather like talking to someone on a telephone, the person at the other end has to fetch something, and puts the handset down on the table, you can tell that the line is still open, but no communication with the other person is temporarily taking place. So prompt.

Therapist:	"Subconscious, it's easy, logical and essential to release Harry, the time has arrived, - that's true too isn't it subconscious?"
Client:	"Yes".

Note: One decision indirectly committing a further decision to be made. It would be illogical, at this stage, for Harry's subconscious to continue to refuse to release him now.

69

Therapist: "Then, subconscious, you carry out that release when I count to three, and click my fingers - one, two, three, click".

(Pause)

Client reacts: Tears come from Harry's right eye, Harry reports that his arm is tingling.

Therapist: "Subconscious, you said that there is another reason for Harry's arm condition does that reason still exist?"

Client: "Yes".

Therapist: "Is it connected with his car accident?"

Client: "Yes!"

Therapist: "Harry wants you to release that reason too, will you do that now?"

Client: "No".

Therapist: "Is it because you are afraid?"

Client: "Yes".

Therapist: "Is it because of the shock of the accident?"

Client: "Yes".

Therapist: "Are you afraid to remember or go back to it?"

Client: "Yes".

Therapist: "But it's over, Harry's perfectly safe in here now, and he is not on his own, and it only takes a moment to release him, and Harry would then be free from it, that's true too isn't it?"

Client: "Yes".

Therapist: "The time has now come for that release too, I'll count to three, click my fingers, and Harry has that wonderful release - one, two, three, click".

Client reacts: Harry momentarily experiences his reaction, both as a physical response and an emotional one. Following the second release, the arm condition can be expected to heal, but, as a supporting back-up, continue.

Therapist: "Subconscious, in a moment, when I ask you to, I want you to carry out a thorough examination of Harry's arm and when you have, say 'yes' once again, subconscious, please carry out that examination now".

(pause)

Client: "Yes".

Therapist: "Subconscious, is that arm now recovering completely?"

Client: "Yes".

<u>Note</u>: A client will be interested in having some estimate of how long that recovery may take, to establish a subconscious estimate, continue using the same hand-holding technique, and proceed as follows:

Therapist: "Subconscious, Harry wants to know how long you estimate it will be, before his arm has recovered enough for him to take up driving again". "In a moment I'll begin to go back over time period names, beginning with months, and I want you to say 'yes' when the time period name is mentioned that is the correct one". "Following that, I'll count back from twelve, and you say 'yes' when I say the number that goes with the time period name, to give your estimated answer". (Slowly) "Months, (pause) weeks, (pause) days?"

Client: "Yes". (days)

Therapist: "Good, now the numbers, twelve, (pause) eleven, (pause) ten, (pause) nine?"

Client: "Yes". (nine)

Therapist: "Subconscious will you confirm that you estimate Harry's recovery will be sufficiently advanced, to allow Harry to drive again in nine days?"

Client: "Yes".

Therapist: "Thank you subconscious".

<u>Note</u>: Phew! Most cases would be much easier.

An additional 'twist' is revealed in the next but simpler

example. In this a lady reported that she was absent-minded over where she had left her reading glasses and was constantly mislaying them. The same arrangements were adopted as in the previous case, and a response established.

Therapist: "Subconscious, are you deliberately causing Mary to forget where she leaves her reading glasses?"

Client: "Yes".

Therapist: "Good, thank you, is there any reason why you do this?"

Client: "Yes".

Therapist: "Does Mary get a benefit from forgetting where she leaves her glasses?"

Client: "Yes".

Therapist: "Is it because Mary doesn't like them?"

Client: "No".

Therapist: "Does Mary feel self-conscious wearing them?"

Reaction: Hesitant, no response.

Therapist: "Is there some similar reason?"

Client: "Yes".

Therapist: "I'll count to three, click my fingers and you tell Mary what that similar reason is then - one, two, three, click".

Client's reaction: Mary smiles, and reports that she just saw the face of her former school friend Ann, but can make no sense of why she had the picture. Mary is pressed to explore for a reason, and remembers Ann wore glasses all the time.

Therapist: "Okay. I'll count to three and click my fingers, and you will see something else about Ann - or just go to another memory - one, two, three, click".

Note: Mary reports remembering seeing Ann with no glasses on one occasion, and then recalls Ann telling her that she never wore her glasses when she went to a job interview. But Mary sees no connection, since she already has a good job.

Therapist: "Subconscious is there some connection with Mary mislaying her glasses, and men in some way?"

Client: "No".

Therapist: "Subconscious, do you know that Mary's glasses are essential to her?"

Client: "Yes".

Therapist: "Then subconscious it would be more convenient if she always knew where she had put them wouldn't it?"

Client: "Yes".

Therapist: "Then will you agree to allow Mary to know why you make her forget where she leaves her reading glasses?"

Client: "Yes".

Therapist: "Then when I count to three, and click my fingers, you tell Mary that reason - one, two, three, click!"

(No reaction)

Note: In some cases, an apparent contradiction between the subconscious agreeing to do something, and then not doing so can arise. The most likely reason to suspect, is that the mind part being dealt with agrees, while another part does not. Rather like the left hand not knowing what the right hand is doing. To resolve such an issue, the objecting mind part must be called to attend.

Therapist: "Subconscious is there some part of the subconscious that objects to Mary knowing, and thereby being freed from her forgetfulness?"

Client: "Yes".

Therapist: "Then have that part come forward and tell Mary what it does for her in her life - what job it looks after".

(pause)

Client: "Protection!"

Therapist: "Subconscious protection part, are you causing Mary's memory lapses with her reading glasses?"

73

Client: "Yes".

Therapist: "Then when I count to three, and again click my fingers, tell Mary what she is being protected from - one, two, three, click!"

<u>Note</u>: Mary says she is thinking of the office in which she works, and suddenly realises consciously, that she is the only one of the five women in her office who wears glasses, even if only for reading, and feels this makes her the odd one out, and less competitive for the promotion she's competing for.

Therapist: "Subconscious, protection part, would you agree that in mislaying her glasses, not only does this cause her inconvenience, but even makes her look less suitable for promotion, because she may appear absent-minded, less efficient and disordered?"

Client: "Yes".

Therapist: "Do you agree that Mary does need to use her glasses?"

Client: "Yes".

Therapist: "Do you also agree that you could protect Mary more, by reminding her where her glasses are, and in doing so make her appear far more efficient?"

Client: "Yes".

Therapist: "Then can I have the attention of the whole subconscious?"

Client: "Yes".

Therapist: "Good, is there any part of the subconscious that still objects to Mary remembering where she puts her glasses?"

Client: "No!"

Therapist: "Good, then I will count to three, click my fingers, and when I do so, please carry out that change - one, two, three click!"

74

Reaction: Mary reports seeing a flash of light in her mind. She is released.

The hand-holding technique is often built into session seven but can also be used earlier even during an initial meeting, and without hypnosis. However, using the technique too early significantly increases the possibility of the subconscious failing to co-operate. This can be particularly true at an initial meeting, where any attempt to use it to bring about change would inevitably result in running straight into an impenetrable barrier, even more so in the absence of hypnosis.

The reason for the reluctance to respond, at an initial meeting, can be understood by comparing the situation to others. Imagine being approached by some total stranger, who demanded of you that you should relate to him details of some highly-embarrassing experience he had heard you had. Alternatively, imagine being approached in a supermarket by someone asking you to lend them five pounds, promising to send it back to you the next day. Most people would be reluctant to do so and prefer the stranger to go away.

However, suppose it was not a stranger but a good neighbour you trusted? If he were to say he needed ten pounds until he got home, when he would return it to you, and if you had it to spare, you would probably be only to happy to help. The comparison is, that we naturally co-operate and respond with those we know more readily than with those we do not, especially when it comes to important personal matters. Similarly in hypnotherapy, trust is built up with repeated sessions which gradually produces increased co-operation.

A situation where the hand-holding technique can be of great benefit, and is likely to enjoy immediate subconscious co-operation, is one where the client reports a condition that could just as equally have physiological causes as psychological ones. Where it is physiological, the subconscious will regard the enquiry as purely a medical matter, and take the same view of the therapists questions as he would with questions by his doctor. So long as the questions remain restricted to the information gathering type, co-operation will continue, but might cease should any attempt be made to suggest change. Nothing can be absolutely guaranteed with this technique, since the questions may be unintentionally misleading or the client's subconscious could misunderstand them, especially the younger the subject is.

Alternatively, the answers given could be on an 'on balance' basis, say 80% yes, 20% no, resulting in a weakened response, perhaps indicating a condition that could be resolved, when some psychological barrier is removed, for instance. However, the subconscious will not attempt to respond to questions by deliberately lying, for lying requires intelligent construction abilities that the subconscious does not have. To cause a person to lie, the subconscious must prompt the conscious mind to do so, and since the hand-holding technique by-passes the conscious mind, that intellectual facility is not available to it. The only recourse the subconscious has if it wishes to lie is for it to simply refuse to co-operate. Indeed, it is the contradiction between the ability to lie by the conscious mind and the not being able to do so by the subconscious that produces the reactions in the 'lie detector'. Where a response is sought and obtained at an initial meeting however, the early proof of the therapist's skill can substantially increase the client's confidence in the therapist, and having impressed him, analysis will get off to a flying start.

The Physiological Idio Motor Response

In this the subconscious is asked to use some bodily part, normally a finger, to signal its replies to questions by physically activating it when the answer is 'yes'. Alternatively, the reaction may be invited to signal 'no'. Some hypnotherapists will employ both hands and ask the subconscious to use one to indicate 'yes' and the other to indicate 'no'. Whilst this form of Idio Motor Response is probably the most widely used method, it suffers from three serious potential problems.

Firstly, the signal may vary in detectability, the degree of movement being directly proportional to the enthusiasm of the subconscious to respond, and this may lead to the possibility of a reply being missed by the therapist which in turn, may run into the problem that the subconscious is reluctant to repeat its response should it be requested to do so.

Secondly, a further potential difficulty is that, by causing the subject to become more aware of a specific finger or other part, meaningless involuntary movements can take place, misleading all, particularly when the intended signals only produce small movements in any case. One only has to observe the tendency for involuntary movements that can occur, when we wish to concentrate on carrying out some important but delicate task: like threading a needle or trying to hold something very steadily while another watches. In fact their are devices that challenge the public to trace a curved wire, carrying a small electric current, with a ring or loop in an attempt not to make contact and light a lamp up, often to be found at fair grounds and very few challengers succeed.

This same involuntary action can also occur with the hand-holding technique, but it is detectable for what it is and is readily distinguishable from any intended 'yes' signal. In this sense the involuntary 'background' signal is a positive asset rather than a nuisance, as it indicates the continuance of the communication. Thirdly, using the finger movement response, the over enthusiastic client may consciously cause any given response to occur. Even when the response is given and is genuine, the client may doubt if it actually came from his subconscious. With the client's confidence possibly being undermined in the process, and lead to the possibility of a complete lack of reliability and co-operation. However, not only is this finger movement method popular with many therapists, some therapist's largely depend on it. On the plus side however, it is useful where only the client and therapist are present during therapy. Naturally, a similar procedure of questioning and negotiating can be adopted as with the hand- holding technique.

Speaking Directly With The Subconscious

This is another amazingly simple technique and one that has three major advantages. Firstly, the technique is not restricted to the yes/no only response. Secondly, where it can be used, i.e., with a client who can grasp this simple knack, it is the easiest technique. Thirdly, it is the fastest technique especially in situations where, using the yes/no approach, negotiations could otherwise prove lengthy or run the risk of over complication. It helps to understand the technique by looking at a fairly common situation, where it often spontaneously occurs, that is in an argument or row which may be triggered by some factor and then become heated.

Where the discourse does turn into a row, and especially when the subconscious is attempting to express its mounting anger or rage, it may well take over the situation and express its emotion. Lacking the intelligent conscious mind's ability for rationality and logic, the subconscious will wish to lash out. Things are said that otherwise would not be, perhaps bad language may be used, doors slammed, items smashed, irrational statements and commitments made and even physical violence ensue. Following the exchange, more often than not, the participants may feel regretful. Alternatively, they may feel that the air has been cleared and in this a positive outcome will have occurred. Whatever the result, most often such people will wonder what came over them, to cause them to react to the degree they had. What happens though, is that the level of subconscious emotion temporarily rises to a point where it overflows the normal barrier of logic and self-restraint, and takes the matter over. By speaking directly with the subconscious a similar procedure is employed, but neither in a confrontational nor an emotional manner. It is as if the barrier which overflowed in the row, is now lowered using hypnosis. A similar situation to the principle of this technique also occurs commonly, for instance we may say something reflecting our subconscious thinking that we had not consciously intended to say. This unintentional vocalisation of thoughts is popularly called a 'Freudian slip'.

An amusing (*to the audience*) example of this, was when the news reader began his report on a French election campaign by saying: "Now a report on the French erection" - subconsciously he was more concerned with the thought of French sexuality in some way. We often say, or let slip something that we believe to be true but then wish we hadn't said it. I once responded to a shop assistant asking me, as I was leaving: "Don't you want your change?", by spontaneously saying "Oh we're terribly rich, and change is such a nuisance". I am certainly not rich, it was my subconscious reflecting my sense of humour, and leaving me to deal with the jokes of the staff as I returned to collect it.

The Method

The subject is told in the conversation to follow that he is to respond without thinking, that is in a spontaneous way he is to say whatever comes to his mind, and without thinking about it first, just as he might in a row.

Next the therapist is to say to the client's subconscious:
Therapist: "Subconscious in a moment I am going to speak to you direct, I want you to take over (*client's name*) voice box, vocal chords and hearing so that when I speak to you, you communicate back to me directly and without (*client's name*) conscious mind playing any part. Subconscious do you understand what it is I ask of you?"

Having a 'yes' the exchange commences. The therapist will, with just a little experience, quickly come to sense if what is said by the subject is actually coming directly from the subject's subconscious. Responses from the subject's subconscious normally tend to be 'snappier' or quicker than might otherwise be the case, to similar questions asked outside of hypnosis and coming from the conscious mind. Certain words will never normally be used by the subject's subconscious. Such words are those indicating indecisiveness such as, possibly, maybe, guess, perhaps, might and the like! During my training the instructor was immensely skilled in this technique, and he would walk among the students who sat in pairs practising it knowing instantly, if what was being said by the students acting the client's role was coming from the subconscious mind or not.

The following case illustrates this amazingly simple yet highly rewarding technique.

The Case of the Weight-Loss Lady

A lady, who had attended for weight-reducing therapy telephoned back a week later to report that it had had no effect. She was invited to attend for a further session to ascertain why. Being just the two of us and needing to discover the reason for the failure of the otherwise normally successful therapy, I decided to use the direct speaking technique. Having told the client how she should respond, I began:

Therapist:	"Subconscious, Jane is very concerned about her weight problem,which seriously hampers her in her hobby even threatening to prevent her continuing with it. Yet you seem not to have taken up the weight loss therapy I gave you. Subconscious, is this because you need more time to bring about weight loss?"
Client:	"No!"
Therapist:	"Do you have some reason for rejecting that change?"
Client:	"Yes".
Therapist:	"What reason do you have?"
Client:	"I don't want to say".
Therapist:	"But subconscious, Jane's weight makes her unhappy and unfit and you are working as a team with her conscious mind, so she's entitled to know your reason isn't she?"
Client:	"Yes".
Therapist:	"Then it makes no sense to hide it from her does it?"
Client:	"No, but she would be hurt". (Notice how she speaks of herself as the third person)
Therapist:	"Conscious Jane, even if you were hurt by it would you still rather know the truth?"
Client:	"Oh Yes I would".
Therapist:	"Good. Subconscious, you have Jane's permission to tell her so will you pass that information to Jane?"
Client:	"Yes".
Therapist:	"Good, so tell her what that reason is".
Client:	"Eric (her husband) comes home drunk and talks

rubbish, he has nasty sexual habits, and he leaves her alone when she's overweight. (Jane opened her eyes) Oh my God, it's true, and I see it all now!" She cried.

Note: I asked her to close her eyes again and go back to direct speaking.

Therapist: "Subconscious, is that the only reason you have to object to Jane losing weight?"

Client: "Yes".

Therapist: "If I could suggest an alternative strategy that would allow her to lose weight, and defend her even better against Eric's unwanted advances would you agree to consider the idea?"

Client: "Yes!"

Therapist: "Good. Suppose, as an alternative to using overweight, which threatens the hobby that gives Jane such pleasure, you were to help her lose weight while, with all the knowledge you have of Eric, you were to build up Jane's confidence and determination. Then she could far more easily fend off those unwanted approaches from Eric, so that in that way Jane has her hobby and does not suffer from Eric's behaviour. Would that be a better idea?"

Client: "Yes".

Therapist: "Does any part of the subconscious object to adopting that new idea?"

Client: "No".

Therapist: "Would it be appropriate to make the changes necessary and bring that new idea into operation in here now?"

Client: "Yes".

Therapist: "Then I'll count to three, click my fingers and you carry out that change in Jane's programming then - one, two, three, click!"

<u>Note</u>: Jane reported herself to be spinning like a top, but knows that she is not. This case was a straightforward situation, not created by a repression, but by faulty self-programming. Albeit, with the best of intentions.

Just Walking In The Rain

The same technique was used in the analytical case to follow, but in session seven. Had it been tried earlier it would most likely not have worked, since rather than the simpler faulty self-programming situation previously quoted, in this case the client's acute agoraphobia was the product of a repression, which had first to be discovered and then released. A further point worth making is that while a client discovering a repressed memory can be expected to be released from its symptom, speaking directly with the subconscious can be used, and often is, as part of that release and to further enhance it.

With the agoraphobic female client, the sessions of analysis had to begin with home visits. Because she was unable to leave her home, or even to go into her garden unless accompanied - even then she suffered considerable anxiety. The usual analytical way of releasing the repression, had proved only partially successful. Switching to the direct speaking technique, the case was to unravel. I asked her subconscious if it had a reason for producing her phobia. It responded with 'Yes'. So the method was proceeded with.

Therapist: "Subconscious, does Andrea know what that reason is in her conscious mind?"

Client: "No".

Therapist: "Subconscious why did you not release her fully, by telling her what that reason is when I counted to three and clicked my fingers?"

Client: "Because she would go out".

Therapist: "Thank you subconscious, but why must she stay in?"

Client: "Because the world is a nasty dangerous place".

Therapist: "Thank you subconscious, but why is the world a nasty dangerous place?"

Client: "Because the neighbour's daughter was murdered, and all the things you hear about on the news".

Therapist: "Subconscious, but everyone goes out, including me, I have travelled to see you, and I am all right. Subconscious, if you saw things as others do, you could get on with life, and go out too, couldn't you?"

Client: "No, because Andrea must be ill".

Therapist: "Subconscious, why must Andrea be ill?"

Client: "Because her family forces her to go outside and if she is ill and in bed they cannot".

<u>Note</u>: Andrea interrupted consciously at this point to say, in a surprised way, that she had recently become mysteriously unwell, and that her doctor was unable to diagnose any cause.

Therapist: "Subconscious, if Andrea felt safe to go out she would not need to be ill to prevent her doing so, would she?"

Client: "No".

Therapist: "So subconscious, will you now agree with my help to develop a plan to allow her to go out?"

Client: "No".

Therapist: "Is there some reason, still not considered, that stands in the way of freeing her?"

Client: "Yes".

Therapist: "Do you know what that reason is?"

Client: "Because she was attacked outside and it would happen again".

<u>Note</u>: Andrea interrupted to explain the minor instance, that she had known of, but until then had forgotten.

Therapist:	"Subconscious is it the combination of the neighbour's experience the incident you just recalled and the news reports that caused you to decide on agoraphobia to keep Andrea indoors?"
Client:	"Yes".
Therapist:	"Is there any other reason?"
Client:	"No".
Therapist:	"Subconscious, if I could suggest a far better way of looking after Andrea would you be prepared to consider it?"
Client:	"Yes".
Therapist:	"Subconscious, suppose you built Andrea up, make her mentally strong gave her great self-confidence and self-assurance, so that she could go out and cope with the world easily, and enjoy life again, would that be a better plan?"
Client:	"Yes".
Therapist:	"Does any part of the subconscious object to that plan?"
Client:	"No".
Therapist:	"Then is it the right time, here and now, to adopt that plan?"
Client:	"Yes".
Therapist:	"Then I'll count to three and click my fingers, and when I do, you do all you need to adopt that new plan completely. - one, two, three, click!"

<u>Note</u>: Andrea reported a sudden jolt in her body.

Before leaving, I told her that I would now expect her to visit me for her last session which she was able to do so and all on her own. At that session, she enthusiastically told me that over the preceding weekend her family had coaxed her to visit a stately home. They had cautiously led her into going outside to view the gardens. One by one, according to their previously-arranged plan, they quietly slipped away from her until she had suddenly found herself on her own in the Lavender garden. With a sudden rush of excitement, she realised she was coping - but not wishing to tempt her luck to desert her - she called out for her family who responded promptly. Session eight passed well and she left.

Just over a week later she rang to tell me of her latest adventure. The family owned a boat which was moored on the Norfolk Broads and to test her further, the family encouraged her to come with them for the weekend. This she did - her first visit in two years. It rained heavily all the first day and with weather prospects seeming no better, it was decided to return home the next morning. Becoming bored with cooped up, she left her family playing cards, and wandered along the bank, excited by her freedom to do so, until her family came eagerly searching for her. "They couldn't believe I had let myself get into the state of being as drenched as I was, but", she said, "pneumonia was a small price to pay for such freedom and pleasure. Amazingly, I didn't even get a cold!"

Spontaneous Handwriting

This method is best used in session four of analysis. The therapist says to the client while he is still in hypnosis: "Before you leave today you will feel a compelling urge, a need, an overwhelming desire to write something down on the paper I give you, what you write is directly related to the cause of your problem. The urge and need is so intense, that you do write that thing down". The same statement is repeated and made immediately before ending the session. Following de-induction and without further exchanges the client is then handed pen and paper. What is written might at first appear obscure or might not, but it is amazing even if with later hindsight, how revealing and relevant what the client writes can be.

Chapter Four

The Induction of Hypnosis
(Self-induction and the induction of others)

Note: In rare cases, the induction of hypnosis can produce a spontaneous abreaction to occur, this can be distressing. Client's and subjects must be made aware of this possibility prior to induction.

From those who are not aware of having experienced hypnosis a wide variety of opinions of it can be expected. Commonly those opinions will be wildly inaccurate. Among such opinions are that the hypnotised person is completely taken over by it; that no memory of the experience will exist; that hypnosis 'zonks' or 'zaps' the person out; and that the person becomes some 'headless' victim of the hypnotic inducer. Often, potential subjects will be much influenced in their thinking by the numerous portrayals of hypnotists as being 'spooky', 'evil', and having 'mystical powers' or 'dominating characters', each hypnotist eager for his next victim. The reality is that, apart from feeling more relaxed, no other sensation is felt! Consequently, at least at first the subject is in for a disappointment at how ordinary they feel. Often complaining that they are not in hypnosis, or erroneously deciding it cannot be induced in them, and in this latter case, deciding it must be because their mind is too strong!

Many people have watched hypnotists perform on stage or screen and saw the hypnotised subjects carrying out actions or performing in a way that makes them appear to be taken over. These performances give a totally distorted picture of the hypnotherapist. The stage hypnotist's subjects act in the way they do because they both expect such reactions to occur and want them to. If they did not the hypnotist would be unable to make them do as they do. As an example of this concept consider the following:

The Failed Experiment

An American university's Department of Psychology reported that a professor had at first thought he disproved the theory that a person cannot be directed in hypnosis, to act against their normal inclinations and behavioural patterns. Finding a female subject appearing to be highly responsive to hypnotic suggestion, it was suggested to her in hypnosis, that upon de-induction, she would immediately become physically aggressive to a selected fellow male student. It was further suggested to her that when the professor clicked his fingers she would feel calm and stop the aggressive response. The experiment was successful and went according to the suggestions. The otherwise placid female, following de-induction and acting quite out of her normal character, began attacking her male student colleague.

In repeated experiments, the same female student was similarly induced to attack other students which she subsequently also did. Finally, she was induced to attack her boyfriend with whom she was known to be deeply in love. Again a similar outcome was to result. Amazed at the success in overturning the previously held theory the professor, somewhat excited by his apparent discovery, thought to test his discovery further. The following morning, amongst the much heightened enthusiasm of everyone, the professor once again induced hypnosis in the same highly responsive female student. He then proceeded to suggest that she again carries out an action, following the de-induction of hypnosis; much in the same manner as he had previously suggested. This time however, instead of becoming aggressive it was suggested she would systematically undress. Immediately the student abandoned the hypnotic trance, opened her eyes and smiled broadly. Somewhat taken aback, the professor asked her why she had reacted in such a way. Still smiling she replied: "Well, I knew I'd be stopped with the aggression before any real harm was done in the earlier experiments, but this time I'm not so sure!" End of failed experiment.

The Hypnotic State

So what is hypnosis, or the hypnotic state? One might equally ask what is meditation? In response, because hypnosis is either similar to or the same as. These are excellent examples of those simple questions that can be very difficult to answer, for even yet, what theories exist, are subjective rather than objective. However, hypnosis is understood in its principles. In the following, I express my own personal interpretations.

Hypnosis is natural and occurs frequently and spontaneously in all of us. 'Miles-away' daydreaming, watching television, listening to music and physically repetitive actions can produce it. Hypnosis is considered by many as a prerequisite state to enter sleep. In itself, hypnosis is entirely harmless, medically, physiologically and psychologically. The hypnotised subject remains completely conscious in the hypnotic state, so too does the subject retain his full control over himself, only acting in a way which is acceptable to him during the experience. The hypnotised subject will remember as much of what takes place after it as he would in a non-hypnotic state. The subject can terminate hypnosis immediately and at his own behest, should he wish to - just as he might terminate daydreaming. The subject can also resist its induction if wished.

Following the induction, the only resultant feeling if any, is of relaxation. However, despite hypnosis being entirely harmless the inducer should be aware of some possible reactions in the subject prior to using the healing techniques. If a feeling of tension or anxiety is felt by the subject upon induction that reaction is not to hypnosis but to some existing hidden subconscious anxiety or tension becoming more consciously evident to him. Such reactions arise because hypnosis reduces the subconscious's ability to suppress anxiety. When a feeling of anxiety results the subject is to be encouraged to continue for the therapeutic objective of the induction is to encourage changes. Such as the release of anxiety through the return of trapped emotions to the intelligent mind, and by the subject re-experiencing them. The subject should not be put off by it for even in feeling such reactions a draining away of them occurs.

Some further points need to be considered. Unless an experience of what is known as a 'spontaneous abreaction' or an 'instant recall' of a previous negative experience occurs, then any anxiety felt on induction will be mild and very easily coped with. Again the anxiety, if felt, will only be like some echo of an earlier negative experience and since the subject clearly survived on that occasion the subject can easily deal with just remembering it. It should be stressed however, that any such reaction of anxiety, upon hypnotic induction, is fairly unusual. In the methods I put forward, no harm can come of the subject because, and I repeat myself, only a memory and not an actual experience occurs. Should a spontaneous abreaction occur in your subject, don't panic, remain calm and comforting and resist any temptation to terminate it unless the subject is medically frail and the reaction more extreme. If you do, you have only done a part job and your subject will almost certainly be worse off. Be reassuring, hold their hand if need be - the experience will last for only about a minute and again, such experiences are very rare. However, in such a situation if you want to see someone amazed, delighted, grateful and enthusiastic just wait two or three minutes more. No experience, in this highly beneficial therapeutic work, can be more satisfying to both subject and therapist than the release of a negative memory whether that release be smaller or larger in its quantity or make-up.

Whilst the recall will definitely be the essence of the moment, over the short-term it will become a 'neither-here-nor-there' matter for the subject. Beware too of resistance, which is the reverse of the spontaneous reaction which will seek to 'protect' the subject from recalling the event. This is because, to it, the memory is an experience that is currently happening, and not some past event, therefore the subject's subconscious may be reluctant to confront it. However, this reluctance is proved unjustified for not only are most repressions outdated by existing conditions, but are also mostly founded upon immature earlier reactions.

What may appear to the subject's subconscious as some awful prospect, instead turns out to be a simple but amazingly good experience and brings with it a permanent benefit. Strangely, at first sight the recall of a pleasant or good memory of an experience has no diminishing effect of the quality of that memory. Indeed, I have experienced great delight in clients who have recalled long since forgotten happy experiences such as recalling taking their first steps in life.

Forearmed by the cautioning points raised, we can proceed with the methods of inducing hypnosis by turning first to self-hypnosis. There are many ways of inducing it. Follow your selected process and then carry out the work you intend. Don't be put off if you feel no difference following the induction procedure because using any of the methods given at their conclusion, the hypnotic state will be present and even if it cannot be felt. With practice, if not initially, sooner or later you will be able to detect its presence. In any case, it makes little difference whether you believe you have been successful in inducing it or not. Just try believing that the sun won't rise in the morning and then check the sky the next day to see if it becomes light. In any case, as suggested, even if you don't feel any effect from the self induction, do the work you intended, following the selected induction routine. Sooner or later you will be in for a pleasant surprise with your results.

A Self-Induction Method

Lying comfortably in bed, first allow yourself the chance to relax. If you can't relax much, begin anyway, for any relaxation prior to self-induction would only have got you off to a slightly better start in any case. Now with your eyes closed, choose an exhalation of breath and mentally label it as a number ten, doing your best to imagine a ten as you do so. However, the lack of visualisation distracts little, should you find this aspect difficult, but it should at least be attempted. Perhaps you could visualise the numbers as if on a door, or a number just floating weightlessly in the air, or some other personal mental visualisation will do.

The better you have this visualisation the slightly more effective the induction is likely to be. After visualising the ten and on the next exhalation, repeat the method above but this time using the number nine. Now continue counting down in the same manner and to include zero. Subsequently begin counting again as before but start counting from nine down to zero again. Following that, of course, count from eight to zero, seven to zero and so on, ending with the final column of one to zero and lastly with a zero itself. Repeat the entire exercise if you want to, but don't be surprised if you do repeat it, to find yourself having drifted off into a pleasant sleep, with the intended work of course, then left undone. Should you have the tendency to drop off to sleep during the first routine, then experiment with shortening it to leave yourself sufficiently awake to use the hypnotic state.

A Second Method of Self-Induction

This technique for self-induction is better used sitting. While sitting comfortably, allow your gaze to fix on some object, say the small light reflecting and shining gently from some spot or surface - a flower, crystal or brass fitting, it doesn't matter what it is so long as it's not intrusive in its own right. Gaze at it steadily, see details and properties in it that you may not previously have noticed. Think of its origins. If mineral, it had its origins in a supernova, the massive natural explosion of a star at least ten times the size of our sun. This rammed and fused elements one into another, and lit up our skies with a light greater than that from all the other stars of the night put together.

Somehow through time, it has journeyed to become incorporated into planet earth, where it was eventually to be formed into its current shape. With all its properties it is now in your room, bathed in the light it now reflects, making it visible. Marvel at it, wonder at it. Its constituent parts are some fifteen billion years old. Now just gaze and think your thoughts of the great wonder to be found - even in something so small, or apparently insignificant. Of course, you might just soak in the object's light or beauty. Whatever your thoughts, just gaze and become absorbed.

After a minute or two, or when you just feel ready, say to yourself, (or think) "I'm going to close my eyes shortly, and when I do, I shall become deeply, deeply relaxed". Repeat this statement two or three times, then simply close your eyes gently. Continue to reflect on your chosen object for a minute or so then proceed with your intended hypnotic state task.

Note: Some people report that looking at a burning candle can produce excellent results. However, there is the question of safety to be considered should the subject then fall asleep.

A Third Method of Self-Induction

Sit, placing the finger tips together, holding the hands around chin height and a little forward from your face and momentarily gaze at them. Then, when ready, repeat three times: "I'm going into hypnosis" follow the third repetition by dropping your hands into your lap and closing your eyes as you do so.

A Fourth Method of Self-Induction

Sit, holding an arm out straight and above one leg. Gaze at a nail on one finger and keep gazing. As you gaze for about one minute, your arm with become heavier and begin slowly to lower. Try to make this lowering process as slow as possible. When the hand has reached and is touching your knee, simply close your eyes.

A Fifth Method of Self-Induction

Another method with wide acclaim is 'clenching and relaxing'. In this, with your eyes closed, you systematically tour the entire body including neck, shoulders, facial, chest and abdomen muscles, together with thigh, leg, foot, arm and hand muscles. Taking each part in a systematic order of your own determination, you first clench or tighten the muscle group holding that tension momentarily while concentrating upon the part. Then relax that part while feeling the relaxation, upon tension release. Again, the method can be repeated. The benefits of this method are both physical relaxation and induced self-hypnosis.

Deepening Self-Induction

Whichever initial method you use, you can deepen it in the following way. Think to yourself, with your eyes remaining closed, "When I move my right hand, I will be twice as relaxed again". Follow this statement with a small gentle, nominal movement of the right hand. Pause, then follow exactly the same procedure with the right foot to be followed by the left foot and left hand in sequence. As you proceed with these nominal movements and following the self-suggestive statement of when I move my (bodily part) say (or think) "I will be twice as relaxed again", this sequence can be repeated several more times.

These self-induction methods of course, can be combined in a way of your own choosing. It is better to experiment to discover what suits you best. For those seeking to induce hypnosis without making any effort, simply watching a psychelitic strobe lamp for a period of ten minutes is extremely effective, as well as being the easiest method of all. This should be done in a dimmed room to heighten its effect. It is essential the rhythm of the light remains constant throughout each induction. There are excellent strobe lamps especially made for this purpose available - the address of a supplier is given in the back of the book.

These lamps are hugely successful in inducing a level of 'quality' hypnosis that can endure the emotion that might be released during therapy. The more professionally active hypnotherapist will find that a strobe lamp makes the induction of hypnosis not only much simpler but very effective too. Personally I always use the strobe lamp with clients even with those that suffer from migraine, although I would temper caution to the less experienced hypnotherapist's and suggest that in such cases they err on the side of caution until more experience has been gained.

Metering Hypnosis

There are meters available which can be used to monitor the hypnotic effect and to register the subconscious tension felt by the client in hypnosis. Should the meter be used - a very simple device, scaled zero to one hundred, subconscious tensions can be registered by it that might otherwise go unnoticed by both the therapist and client.

The meter is connected to the client by a wire which leads to two sensors contained within a band that is placed around one of the client's hands. An unfelt tiny electrical charge from a small battery, registers the varying electrical resistance between two discs touching the palm. The change in the electrical resistance, caused by variations in the moisture on the palm is then detected on the meter.

The procedure can be reduced to an extraordinary simplicity. Initially, prior to the hypnotic induction, the meter is adjusted so that it registers half-way up the scale, i.e., at fifty. As the hypnotic induction takes effect, the meter will drop to about forty. If, instead it rises, then tension in the subconscious is being felt, although the induction is still proceeding. Assuming that the meter records a reading of approximately forty, hypnosis can be assumed, particularly if this follows the client having watched a psychelitic lamp for ten minutes.

As the work proceeds, the therapist should look at the

readings from time to time and write them down in the margin of his notes. Where the readings become higher, say at sixty or more, the client should be encouraged to continue with the topic that has caused them for higher readings reflect subconscious anxiety.

At the end of each session, the readings are then added together and the sum total divided by the number of readings recorded to give an average result. For instance, say fifteen recordings have been noted and their sum total amounts to approximately twelve hundred, then the average becomes eighty. As the sessions continue, the average should steadily fall until eventually, an average of forty or less is achieved.

During the last session the therapist can then go back over his notes, and once again raise the issues which produced the previous higher readings, but observe the meter as he does so. If, as is normal, there is virtually no reading above forty, some independent evidence exists that the earlier anxiety has been drained away, with the client's subconscious now appearing indifferent to the matters.

Three disadvantages can be encountered with the meter aid: if the client is restless he may, by pressing his hand down, artificially decrease the electrical resistance and produce higher but misleading readings; secondly, should he have to interrupt the session - to go to the toilet for instance, the meter cannot be used for the remainder of the session, because there can be no accurate way of knowing what effects the interruption has had, or at what setting the meter should be adjusted to; and thirdly, in some cases, the client's hands may be so dry that with the small electrical charge available, no beneficial reading can be obtained. However, where this last problem arises, the application of some handcream can assist, giving some twenty or thirty minutes for recordings to be taken. (The address of the supplier of these meters is also given in the back of this book.)

The Induction of Hypnosis in Others
(The Hand Shaking Induction)

Other than the lamp technique, hypnosis can easily be induced in another by physical or oral means. Of course, you may also invite the subject to induce hypnosis in themselves by using one or more of the self-induction techniques mentioned earlier.

One method, other than either using self-induction or a light source, is to make a small mark on the palm of your right hand and hold your hand about 40cm from the subject's eyes, your palm turned towards them. Then say: "In a moment I shall bring my hand down towards your eyes and as I do so, look at my hand using this mark - indicating the mark on the palm, with your left hand - as your focal point. When my hand is close to your eyes, it will glide down in front of your nose, lips and chin. When my hand glides down past your eyes, just close your eyes and keep them closed".

The statement is spoken softly and unhurriedly. Next, having carried out the action, say: "In a moment I shall pick up your right hand; don't help me at all, just let it remain floppy and loose". Then gently, while standing to the right of the subject, take the right hand and lift it about 25cm and gently rock it from side to side, say 15cm towards yourself, then back 30cm towards the subject - that is a 30cm arc swing is made.

Continuing to repeat this gentle movement and then say softly: "In a moment, I shall count to three, and then drop your right hand into your lap, and when I do, you will be amazed at how much more relaxed you become. Here we go". Next count aloud to the rhythm of the three side-to-side hand movements - as described, and on the count of three, allow the hand to fall into the subject's lap. Move to the subject's left side, saying: "I'm coming round to take your left hand". When on the subject's left, repeat the exercise as for the right hand. It is a good idea to repeat the exercise, on a first occasion with a subject, because it is quite likely that the subject may have concentrated more on what you have been doing, than simply allowing the induction of hypnosis to happen. Moreover, once the subject is more relaxed about what is to take place to induce hypnosis, the subject will just let it happen. This induction is enough in itself for hypnosis to be sufficiently deep for work to commence. Flickering eye lashes and a slight change of the subjects posture or pallor are all good indications of a successful induction. It must be stressed that when a subject has his eyes closed, the therapist should never, ever touch the subject without him previously being informed of the intention. For instance, don't just suddenly place your hand on his shoulder while saying "relax, let your shoulders drop" or similar.

Also, take care never to bump into them or accidentally knock them. Certainly never let your hand touch them or their hair when passing it close to their eyes and face during the hand pass. Note too that a nose protrudes. If you do cause an unplanned or unannounced physical contact, even a slight one, trust in you by your subject will be reduced, and the greater the physical contact the greater the reduction of trust will be, for they will just be waiting for the next accident. However mistakes and misjudgements can occur, and if they do you will need to apologise and reassure them - it is rather a damage limitation exercise. However, in doing so, take care not to make too much of the incident.

An Oral Technique

In this method you merely talk your subject into hypnosis and the following will serve that purpose well. Please note however, no artificial voice projection should be used, just a gentle slowly paced, quiet presentation is best.

The Script

(*Name*) Please gently close your eyes, and just let them stay closed. (*Name*) Shortly, very shortly you will begin to feel deeply and peacefully relaxed. Those feelings of relaxation are already beginning, and continue to bring an inner harmony to your mind. These feelings bring with them a sense of peace, and tranquillity, so that you feel more and more relaxed. As you continue to relax and relax, you feel good.

As you become more and more at ease, it doesn't matter if at times, you find your mind just wandering away to some pleasant thought, because your inner mind continues to listen and enjoys the growing sense of peace, harmony and tranquillity that is growing and developing within you now. (*Name*) You know those wonderful feelings you can have when sleeping soundly, how you sometimes feel that you wish that you could just be left to doze and slumber, you remember how you felt, lazily laying on a lawn - or some beach in the sun, perhaps drifting in and out of a dozing sleep, yawning and just wanting to stay where you were. In a moment, I shall count slowly back from ten and go all the way down to zero. As I do, you find that you relax more and more with each number I count, until just as you've felt on those lazy occasions in the past, you feel deeply and beautifully relaxed once again, and as I count down I want you to feel yourself going down into calmness.

Ten, feeling more peaceful; nine, relaxing more and more; eight, just keep gently listening to my voice; seven, breathing more deeply and breathing more slowly; six, becoming calmer and calmer; five, becoming sleepier; four, just lazily drifting; three becoming even more and more relaxed; two, feeling as if you could just doze off into a deep and beautiful sleep; one, feeling calmer and calmer, more and more at peace; and zero, now totally relaxed, totally at peace. As you continue to listen to the sound of my voice,

I want you to have a thought simply drift into your mind, just picture yourself looking into a beautiful night's sky, and there in the distance seeing a solitary silver blue star, one solitary star, millions and millions of miles away. Just one tiny dot of light twinkling away. As you look at that star you are becoming ever more, and more relaxed. You feel good, you are becoming ever more peaceful. As you do, just keep that tiny silver blue star as a picture in your mind, and soon very, very soon you will find that you just drift off into a deep and beautifully feeling of peace and tranquillity, and as you do I'm going to count down from ten, and go all the way to zero again as you continue to relax even more and more.

Just continue to listen to the sound of my voice, as you find yourself becoming sleepier and just drifting. From time-to-time you may find yourself almost dropping off to sleep, because you feel so peaceful, so at ease, so calm and relaxed and each number I say, is like a step deeper down into tranquillity, a step down into harmony and an inner peace, now we begin. Ten, deeper down. Nine, just letting go. Eight, relaxing and feeling good. Seven, calmer and quieter, more and more peaceful. Six, deeper and deeper down into peacefulness. Five, feeling more silent and still inside. Four, feeling sleepy. Three, nearly all the way down now. Two, soon completely relaxed. One, down into total calmness and relaxation. Zero, now totally relaxed.

(Name) There's no such thing as a hypnotised feeling, just a sensation of peace and harmony, and you are enjoying those good feelings now. Sometimes there are other pleasant feelings in hypnosis; some people feel a sensation of heaviness, or a lightness instead. These feelings may exist only in the arms or legs, but sometimes they may be felt all over or, change from one sensation to another. Sometimes a pleasant gently tingling can be felt, but always there are feelings of harmony, relaxation, peace, tranquillity, and inner quietness, and you feel them now. Good feelings, wonderful feelings, (Name) Shortly I'm going to help you, and as you relax even more and more, you find that your inner mind responds and participates in a fulfilling and satisfying way that delights you, as you begin to free yourself to become your true self - all feelings and ideas that you want to have and grow to enjoy more and more.

The Eye Induction Method

Hypnosis can be induced in another way, but a way I never use myself. Invite the subject to look into your eyes without blinking. You then appear to the subject to be looking back into his eyes without blinking yourself. Only the technique used is whilst appearing to look back into his eyes, your gaze is actually fixed on his forehead instead. While suggesting from time to time that he tries, implying the possibility that he may not be able, to resist blinking before you do. He then tries not to blink. If he fails, as he will do, you invite him to make a further attempt of beating you by being the last to blink. When, as is inevitable, he has blinked first after three or four attempts, reassuringly invite him to relax, close his eyes and keep them closed. Proceed if necessary to deepen the hypnotic induction you will have produced. It is a variation of this induction method, that gives rise to the saying: "Look into my eyes", that is so frequently heard of in connection with hypnotists. Since we are concerned with hypnotherapy and healing, such 'tricks' are not recommended, and the explanation of it is put forward more in an academic sense.

Deepening Hypnosis in Another

Sitting at the subject's side, proceed softly and leisurely by saying:

"With your eyes remaining closed, I'd like you to begin to imagine yourself becoming lighter and lighter. Becoming lighter and lighter, until (pause) like a child's balloon at a fairground, you imagine yourself as if you are beginning slowly and gently to float up from the chair (pause) floating in the room, say 'yes' when you are floating in the room".

(Await 'yes') "Okay! Now just keep feeling that lovely feeling, it's just like the pictures you see of astronauts, floating weightlessly in space. Now, I want you to imagine yourself nearing the ceiling. (pause) Imagine putting your hand out to bounce gently off it but finding that, without any sensation of contact, your arm just goes through it followed by the rest of your body (pause) so that you find yourself weightless and in the room above. Say yes when you are there. (pause) (Yes!) Now feel yourself weightlessly, effortlessly, floating on up until you float out of the building and into the air outside. Say 'yes' when you are outside. (pause) (Yes!) Now see yourself gently floating/moving away. Look at the scene below".

Note: At this junction make some suggestions with a few seconds apart, of what they might see. Suggest as if they were taking snapshots of the things over which they pass then keep helping with suggestions of town or countryside images.

Continue by saying: "I want you to keep going now until you see in the distance, the facade of a large stately home in the country. Say yes when you see it. (pause) (Yes!) Now float gently towards it and when you arrive come down to land, very, very softly and gently, until you are standing on the large stone terrace in front of it. Say yes when you're standing on the terrace. (pause). (Yes!)

Continue: "In a moment, when I ask, I want you to feel yourself walking across that stone terrace, and down the five stone steps which lead down to the big beautiful green lawn - feel the sensations of walking as you go. Now see yourself do that, and say yes when you are standing on the edge of the soft green lawn

103

(pause) (Yes!) To your left is a beautifully carved stone vase, full of beautiful flowers in perfect blossom and bloom. Just glance at it now, and tell me what colour or colours do you most notice? (pause for reply) Now look to your right, and tell me what colour, or colours do you notice in the vase standing there?

(Pause for reply) (Note the purpose of the colour questions is given in the chapter on analysis.) The entire process, from hand passing to the conclusion with the vases, should take about three minutes or so. Naturally, some subjects respond better to some methods of induction, than they do to others.

However, you will surprise yourself with your results - especially with a little practice.

An Alternative Method of Deepening

Following the previous method, or the hand-passing technique by itself, a further deepening of the hypnotic state can be obtained by using another method.

Say to the subject: "In a moment with your eyes remaining closed, I want you to count down from ten to zero but in a rather special way. Imagine each number in your mind before you say it out loud and then, between each number you first imagine and then say - and as if you can feel it happening as you say it, say deeper and deeper asleep, okay? Do you understand what I want you to do?"

Explain again if the subject does not. "Okay, then call the numbers out". When the subject says 'zero', say to him: "Now, with your eyes remaining closed, bring that zero back on to the screen of your mind and hold it there. Say yes when you have". (pause). (Yes!) Continue: "Now I'll count to three, click my fingers and that zero will just disappear - watch it go. One, two, three, click! Has it gone? (pause) (Yes!) Repeat the counting to three and click your fingers again if the zero remains. This procedure, used with a subject already in an hypnotic state, can be expected to take him into what is known as the 'somnambulistic' level of hypnosis.

Other Techniques
The Five to Zero Technique

The method lends itself well to such experiences as childbirth, dental treatments and similar situations, that call for little intellectual contribution from the subject, and where relaxation would help. It is also particularly useful in dealing with sudden shock. The technique can be used on its own or in conjunction with suggestion scripts to support them. Indeed, it was this technique that the lady referred to in the extract from the letter to be quoted in Book Three, chapter three, when reporting her childbirth experience.

The Five to Zero Technique in Application

The subject simply counts down from five to zero while attempting to picture the numbers as he does. Initially, the speed of counting may be as fast as is desired, but it should gradually be slowed if commenced at a fast rate. Eventually a rhythm should be aimed for where each number occurs as the subject exhales. The numbers must be repeated over and over again; they, and nothing else is important.

The numbers must be forced into the conscious mind if necessary and become the dominant commanding point of attention. Everything else is secondary and inconsequential. This technique can quickly induce a state of relaxation and calmness.

De-Induction

Following, the induction of hypnosis and any therapy that is carried out, de-induction is essential if the subject is then to return to normal activity. De-induction can be easily achieved by using the following script: "In a moment, I'm going to ask you to return to the here and now and then to open your eyes. When you do so, you will continue to remain calm and beautifully relaxed, but be vigilant and alert so that you can do what you need to do, like driving and walking, and all in the way you normally would. Now, when you are ready, come back to the here and now, and then when you have, open your eyes please".

Repeat the same message, should the subject be enjoying the hypnotic experience and is reluctant to come out of it. In all my work, I have never experienced any difficulty or problem with de-induction, save for one occasion. In this instance, a wealthy female client refused my suggestion, reporting herself feeling too nice to accept it, and said she would happily pay the fees of my remaining clients of the day because she was feeling so good. So much for the fears of those never having experienced professionally-induced hypnosis! Should you have induced hypnosis in yourself, a similar statement to the one given above, either thought or expressed will happily serve the same purpose.

It is interesting to speculate on how the mind has such very different capacities in hypnosis when compared to the non-hypnotic state. My own theory is that, and directly proportional to the degree that hypnosis exists in the subject, two main possibilities arise. Firstly, (and there can be little doubt of this) the otherwise natural barrier between the subconscious and conscious minds is lowered or reduced. Secondly, the mind's capacity to transmit and exchange memories, emotions, thoughts and reactions within itself is increased, either by reducing the electrical resistance to such transmissions or because in hypnosis, the mind experiences a heightened electrical discharge. Of the two, I feel it more likely to be the heightened electrical discharge that creates the increase in mental transmissions and exchanges. Certainly the increase in electrical discharge could account for the commonly reported state of feeling 'washed-out' by subjects, following a particularly active session - the result, as it were, of using up resources to produce that electricity.

A comparison might be made with a battery being subjected to a temporary heavy loading. However, any washed-out feeling, unlike physical tiredness, normally soon recedes. Whatever does happen hypnosis allows us, even more when worked on by another, to tap into that detailed memory of life that we all have. Added to these possibilities is the fact that the more we deliberately experience the state the better the results tend to become. In the hypnotic state, we can even recall events occurring during sleep or unconsciousness. The following is an intriguing illustration of this principle and of the limited intellectual resources of the subconscious.

The Case of the Unconscious Lady

A young lady came to me, reporting she not only had a phobia of roads which she could only cross if escorted, but had to walk on the path as far from the roadside as possible. Even then, she reported she had to touch fixed objects like walls, railings and buildings as she proceeded. She was consciously aware of an experience she once had, and which she thought was the origin of her condition. She explained that when she was ten years old, she crossed a wide empty road with her grandmother, and in the middle of the road, her grandmother collapsed. The girl shouted for help while remaining at her grandmother's side, but her calls went unheeded. With the stress of the situation mounting, she eventually collapsed, having fainted. (Fainting in this way, can be the illogical attempt by the subconscious to help the victim blot out an unacceptable emotional situation, so as to protect the conscious from further pain). The usual method of analysis was undertaken, and although it proceeded well brought virtually no change of any significance.

Since she had previously recalled coming round quite soon after fainting, it had been easy during analysis to make the mistake of thinking that the alarming incident itself was at the root of her problem, and that her abreaction of it would release her from her phobia in the usual way. However, this was not so - the conventional approach failed and something was missed.

Knowing that the subconscious continues to react and record, even during an unconscious state, I decided to explore the memories of that brief period of unconsciousness specifically. In the analysis, the subconscious did not make the deduction that any such information was connected with our quest. For my part, no indication was given that it was during the fainting condition, that the phobias were laid down. In any case, such a situation is very rare. When her subconscious was specifically requested to reveal its thoughts after she had fainted, she spontaneously exclaimed: "Grandmother is dead and I shall be run over and be dead too". The interpretation was: you can collapse on the road and die or be killed.

Despite her grandmother surviving the incident and the client having no other negative road experiences, the self-programme had remained. The thoughts it produced were gradually reinforced, when subsequently crossing roads. Knowing of her subconscious thoughts, negotiation with her subconscious could proceed and which finally resolved her condition. This last case has been included in this chapter on hypnosis, because it is an interesting example of the unusual and because it illustrates how essential hypnosis is for resolving such cases. Without hypnosis I believe the resolution may never have occurred, and would have led to goodness knows what, for the lady was in a highly neurotic condition when she first attended for analysis and only twenty one years old at that time.

Chapter Five

Conducting an Analysis

What has been set down so far, has now brought us to the exciting and satisfying situation where your knowledge can be put to practical use. We now begin the journey from theory to practice with all the amazing consequences of success that can be expected as a result. However, some points should be considered prior to that final transition. You may be using this series of books to help yourself, help another as part of your knowledge as a professional hypnotherapist or to assist you in some other profession. Alternatively, you may merely have bought the books out of curiosity in order to seek a greater insight and understanding of the human condition. With so many possible uses I will assume, for simplicity's sake, that you are going to use this knowledge in the role of a hypnotherapist, whether professionally or not. Conscientiously conducted hypnotherapy, along the lines to be set out, can do much good.

Treatment however, once started, must be continued with until the symptoms have been resolved or terminated only following an extended attempt, where little or no progress has been achieved and continuation offers little apparent prospects. Inevitably, some percentage failure rate will occur. However, since the success rate from the therapy techniques given is high, you should be expecting at least an 85% success rate even from the outset.

Where success eludes you following conscientious therapy, it must be the client and not yourself who has caused that outcome. If the same dedication is applied to all you work with, and that dedication works with some nine out of ten, then logic must have it that, in the case of the tenth client he, rather than you have brought that result about in some way. In my experience, among such people are those who lack commitment. For instance, everything else rather than their appointment has priorities, with them rearranging appointments readily perhaps seeing their attendance more as an inconvenience. So too are problems more likely where little or no financial commitment is made by the client, though this is less relevant among family and friends.

However, following the analysis methods set out, you will be seen to have made a genuine effort so the client can do little to criticise the therapy. In all my years as a professional hypnotherapist, I have never been confronted by a dissatisfied client asking for the return of his fees or claiming that I have let them down. Sometimes the client's subconscious will deliberately seek to disrupt or terminate treatment.

Watch out for the client who is often too ill to attend, or the client who interrupts sessions to enquire if the therapy is getting anywhere or starts to throw doubts, not onto the therapist but the general nature of the treatment, or repeatedly expresses the view that the therapy will not work for him. In very rare cases, where the need of the subconscious to protect the client from resolving his problem by confronting it, is strong enough, it will invent a reason. With its lack of intelligence, such a termination of treatment in the presence of the therapist, can be bizarre in the extreme. Their invented reason makes sense to them, but is absurd to the therapist.

The Book and Fee-Throwing Lady

I once had a lady who suddenly got up from the couch, went to my bookcase, extracted a book and threw it down on my desk saying:

"If you're so clever why do you need all these books, and if you're not clever why am I paying your fees?". She then threw her fee for the session onto my desk and walked out. During all of this I said nothing but merely observed, for clearly she had come to the point of a subconscious crisis. She knew she needed to confront the unacceptable truth in herself, if she continued. Anything I could have said would be used against me. The best hope was that she should see the folly of her actions, and this she did.

Most apologetically she rang for a further appointment during which time, we discussed her previous reaction which she readily agreed had been her subconscious resistance to therapy, and even admitted that what she had been prompted to seek, was a confrontation with me to end our professional relationship. The case was to be satisfactorily resolved in the two sessions that followed. If you conduct yourself in a natural way, appearing to have no particular views or opinions, are courteous, kind, sympathetic, non-critical, reassuring, giving little or no actual advice, have reasonable accommodation to work from and be of tidy appearance, then no fault exists in the therapist for the subconscious resistance to latch on to.

The Case of the Angry Lady

I have never felt threatened by a client, even given the amazing mental state that some people arrive in. On one occasion a lady entered my office, and after exchanging greetings I invited her to sit down. Suddenly she changed and became a trembling body of rage and while swearing profusely, she stood leaning on my desk, looking straight at me claiming that she would not do as I said because she was fed up with being told what to do. "I've come here to tell you what to do, you are going to listen to me, nobody else does". Crying, shouting and displaying anger at the world in general, for what it had done to her, she continued until the session time was over. All I did was to make the minimum of responses. Eventually and tactfully I brought the session to a close. I was amazed to hear her coolly and politely arrange her next appointment with my wife.

At the second session, although she reacted much less intensely, it ran much the same as the first one. During the third session with her anger considerably lower, I was able to persuade her to sit down, and allow hypnotherapy to commence, the first two sessions themselves having been therapeutic for her of course. This otherwise greatly intimidated female had become so desperate to hit back from a position of security, that she was prepared to pay my fee, just to satisfy her anger. I really believe that, had I not let her have her way, insisting for instance that I was in charge, then the exercise would have failed.

My response to the client who shows resistance, or reacts in some unexpected way is always to be quiet, sympathetic, calm and tolerant. Not reactions borne of timidity but from the strength of genuine care and empathy. Even in their states of psychological torment they can perceive and recognise genuineness, and under such circumstances a greater feeling of trust will emerge. They have mentally attacked the therapist in some way and the therapist has not responded in a critical, defensive or commanding way as they most probably expected. They have become safe with him; they can be themselves and work can begin.

The message I wish to convey, is that firstly be professional and secondly, don't expect neurotic people to behave rationally. However I must re-emphasise that in what I have just said, I have referred to the very, very rare exceptions - not the norm! Indeed I only refer to these instances to arm you, because sod's law states that early on in your work as a hypnotherapist, you will meet just such a client and one who might otherwise have put you off, and that would have been a shame and a great loss. The benefits you will bring to humanity will have to be experienced to be believed and as I say, not least by yourself.

Session One

The client has arrived and as most do, urgently needs reassuring. The client will almost always be apprehensive of you, himself, hypnosis and the methods you will be using. He will only have hearsay and the stage hypnotist to go on. He is only with you because he is desperate. He has probably tried everything else and all failed! You are his last resort while actually you were his first. The client does not expect to be cured, but he has to try. In the more extreme cases, he will take the view that he doesn't know what he has let himself in for but desperation has forced his hand. He is with you and initially, probably at least mildly terrified, even regretting he came. He has worked out what you will do to him and what will happen and he doesn't much care for the prospect. He would almost as soon leave as stay. To him, by arriving he has 'done it', God help him, for he has only himself to blame. Hopefully he has read this particular series of books, your leaflet, or come by recommendation for if he has he will feel easier.

For my part, I dress informally and display a cheerful confidence while being attentive, courteous, kind and sympathetic. My priority is to put him at ease as quickly as possible. I reassure clients by saying such things as: "There is nothing to the sessions as all we do is talk. The sessions are easy and enjoyable" If the person is in a highly emotional state, I interrupt my normal routine of first seeking details of them and instead, take them into hypnosis and either sit with them and encourage them to tell me about their problem, or carry out my normal introduction process while they are more relaxed in hypnosis. Additionally, I am perfectly happy should they seek the comfort, as many do, for them to have someone with them. I shall want to know their marital or boy/girl-friend status. Do they have any children? What is or was the construction of the family they grew up in? Do they have, or have they had, sleep problems such as repeating dreams, nightmares, sleepwalking or talking in their sleep? What do they do for a living? What do they want me to call them - they may have presented themselves as Michael but prefer to be called Mike. I ask for details of any medication they may be taking which at an appropriate time, I shall look up, for not only can their medication give some insight of their doctor's understanding and approach, but also help to separate from his symptoms any adverse effects that the client might be experiencing from his prescription.

Although I will probably know before his arrival the nature of his problem, or it will be mentioned early in our initial meeting I usually leave going into the details of it until I have the other information I need. There are several reasons for this. Going into detail of their condition can often bring about emotional reactions, instantly hampering me to gain a background, before plunging headlong into what might then have to be the start of the therapy, thus leaving me to treat a client I know little or nothing about. In such a situation, confusing information can pour out in a torrent, leaving the therapist confronted with a tangle of detail. As an example, the client with relationship problems may present a list of disjointed and disastrous experiences with previous partners, leaping from one to the other - of course, while expecting the therapist to keep track.

Any misunderstandings or errant conclusions the therapist makes as a result of attempting to follow him, may be seen by him as the therapist not understanding or following him. Another reason for leaving symptom details until later, is that I shall want him to take a Leusher colour test. He can't do that if I have raised his emotional state by going into the details of his problem, to a level where hypnosis has to be induced. There again, he will have questions he needs to ask, and you will also need to explain the procedures ahead and reassure him regarding hypnosis, etc. You don't really want to be forced to induce hypnosis in the client before you have set the ball rolling if you can help it. Sometimes it is necessary, but I always feel that when hypnosis has to be induced as a priority, both parties are pitched in at the deep end. Fortunately, and despite what has been said, the client may not only want to but also be able to discuss his problems rationally. Indeed this is mostly the case. However, I try to stick to my formula for the first session as far as I can, since the logical sequence reduces the risk of important information being overlooked.

My preferred routine in the first session, particularly with the more rational client, is to greet the client and put him at his ease, and then to ask for a brief indication of what he is attending for. Following this I seek out his background, carry out a Leusher colour test and then return to his symptoms for further details. Of course, during this process I answer the client's questions as they are presented. Next I explain what I expect of him.

When it does come to dealing with his symptoms I go into some detail such as asking when did it start? Did anything significant happen in the two years preceding its onset? (You will recall that a repression can remain hidden, until some other emotional situation is experienced, and that this secondary effect can bring into action the original repression. This having occurred, the emergence of the symptom can take from a day to up to two years to appear.) I probe this period in depth. Sometimes the client will be insistent that this secondary experience is the cause of his problem, and the be-all-and-end-all of it too.

Where this belief is firmly held by the client, watch out for him expecting treatment to be specifically directed at it - a prerequisite of the 'are we getting anywhere' questions. I explain that a secondary situation often brings to light an earlier repressed experience and it is this that requires identifying and resolving. Following this explanation, I hope to gain his willing co-operation in releasing that repression. This explanation is often necessary in such cases, because the client will frequently say that such and such occurred prior to the emergence of his symptom, but then claim either that he has dealt with it, or that it is irrelevant because it was a happy experience: like being promoted, marrying, etc. On some occasions, a client will claim that what he needs is to be 'zonked out' and told to 'pull himself together'. The client will expect the therapist to go into details of his symptom because to him, as mentioned before, it has become the dominant thing in his life. However, as was also stressed earlier, any protracted discussion of his symptoms will hardly be of much benefit.

The client needs to understand that the resolution of his problem is to be found in its cause, not the symptom itself, which is only the result. The client needs to understand that to do this, he must commence the process by using 'free association', which I explain to him. It is also important to ask the client what he has done about his problem, for he may have been to a hypnotherapist before and subsequently hold erroneous views in what he expects of you. He may have been to a psychiatrist had operations or made several other attempts to resolve his plight. All of this information is always written down, and gives a considerable insight of your client before you proceed. Of course he expects you to show an interest in him and ask questions, so feel no reluctance in asking. Sometimes, especially where any doubt may exist that his problem could be resolved, I use the hand holding technique.

The hand-holding technique can be most useful as well as

reassuring and pleasantly surprising to the client, giving an early boost to his confidence in the therapist. Following all this I sit the client down and get him to relax into hypnosis, using the strobe light that I mostly use for hypnotic induction. While he is looking at the lamp I will ask any further questions that are appropriate and/or deal with any further points he raises.

For what remains of the first session, following the information exchange and the induction of hypnosis, I prompt the client to talk to me about himself and his life's experiences, often beginning by asking him about his earliest memories. In the process of free association, the client must be encouraged to say not only what he wants to say, as if as a relief like that from a confession, but everything else that comes into his mind, even if it is disagreeable to him, seems unimportant, illogical, irrelevant or is a repetition of what has been said before. Even if it seems ordinary, uneventful or something he clearly knows about anyway. In fact the benefit of free association is so enormous that by using this method only, can amazing results be produced. Indeed, it's the method recommended by one of the largest associations of hypnotherapists in Europe!

For those readers seeking a less demanding analysis approach, nothing will be lost in trying eight sessions of free association, as opposed to the method otherwise recommended. However, should free association alone be used, there is always a possibility that 'transference' may occur and when it happens with a client, he may transfer his feelings onto the hypnotherapist and much in the way he transferred his feelings to his mother and with all the complications that may have caused. Whilst this consideration is of little importance with clients that are only temporarily connected to the therapist during analysis, it is more important with relatives and friends. However, this potential complication becomes virtually negligible when free association is limited to the first four sessions of analysis. Additionally, it's much easier for clients to talk about themselves over only four sessions, rather than over eight, even then they may feel they have little of importance worth saying. Fortunately, many clients will take to the idea with enthusiasm and happily talk away. This is of course excellent, both for the client and therapist, for when the client is enthusiastically talkative, he is off to a terrific start.

At least as often however, the client is reluctant to talk much and where this happens, I point out how essential it is that he should participate through talking, by explaining to him it doesn't matter what is talked about because through talking, he will give me information that he may not even realise will help me. Not only that but talking about anything in hypnosis will exercise his mind in a way nothing else can equal, preparing his mind for the different work that comes later.

I also point out that in so doing, his subconscious will learn that it can trust me. This is because, unlike normal experiences, I shall not offer advice, criticise, judge him, think him silly, tell him he's wrong, inadequate or suggest that he pulls himself together. Instead I shall listen with interest and because of that, trust will develop to the point where I can ask his mind to bring about change.

Lastly, I explain that in the course of free association, the root cause of his problem will begin to move nearer to his conscious threshold, making it much easier to release. I sometimes illustrate this last benefit, by comparing it to the situation of a table tennis ball, hidden in a tub of corn. "You don't know where the ball is, but as you move the corn the ball, being so much lighter, will bit by bit move towards the surface". (It is this factor that makes a premature termination of treatment unwise, because the symptom or the anxiety may become more pronounced). Even with the explanations, the client may be reluctant to talk. If he is, I shall prompt him by asking questions about his earliest memories. How did his school life go? What about his early family life, his Christmas and holiday experiences and the like.

Naturally, his chosen subject will often be his symptoms and in which case I will let him carry on, since unlike the earlier situation, that is when initially talking to him to gain a background of him he is now in hypnosis and anything may be talked of. Subsequently, in talking about his symptoms and without his realising it he is already beginning to release them. Remember, this is because the first session and that other rules apply in subsequent sessions, in which, should he fail to 'burn himself out' of talking about his symptoms, he will need to be encouraged to talk more of other subjects. In any case, symptom discussion should be restricted to the first two sessions. However there is a difference between his discussing the symptom itself, and his talking of his personal history in which it has played a role as experiences.

If the client wants to continue along the lines of repeatedly saying what they were or are doing to ease their symptoms, complaining that nobody understands; asking if you do; or saying they can't ever see themselves getting better, then this is symptom discussion. Alternatively he may repeatedly say what an awful problem it is for him, what he can't do but would like to, or he may begin speculating and intellectualising about his symptoms, analysing it, all this too, is really symptom discussion.

If, on the other hand, the client goes through the details of his life by talking about how his symptom effected his experiences one way or another, that is good therapeutic free association, and can be allowed to form even the bulk of the work done in the first four sessions. However, it will be far better if the equivalent of at least one session is allocated to other topics and memories.

In free association the therapist should only speak when he

really has too. Ninety per cent of the time it is the client who should be talking, while the therapist writes down, as best he can, all that is said.

You may find it useful to develop your own shorthand. M for mother, ch for child, sch for school, st for something or sometimes, ng to represent the negatives; no good, awful, terrible, failed, hated, etc. For example: "rem D took me jnr sch, sch ng never liked it. D. ng attitude to me st". In full, that would mean to me: "I remember Dad taking me to junior school, I never liked school. Dad had the wrong attitude to me, sometimes".

Writing down what your client says has four benefits. One, almost always in the first few paragraphs the client will, without realising it, refer directly or indirectly to the cause of his problem or at least, give some clue. Two, you have a visible record of what was said and one you can scan or look back to readily. I never use a tape recorder in free association because the client may well feel inhibited by it, and be less inclined to talk about highly confidential and personal information, while being recorded.

If it is written down, goodness knows under what circumstances, he could refute he had ever said such a thing. Three, you can read it, or part of it, back to him in a subsequent session and help him pick up where he left off in the previous one. Another advantage is that you can mark off points of interest that might be important later, and this cannot be so easily done with a tape recording. Four, writing down what he says will keep you concentrating, because there could be little worse for the client/therapist relationship than your client talking away, only to find that you had let your mind wander and had not taken a word in for some time. Lastly, you may need the information should the client revisit you even years later.

At all times be prepared with tissues and sympathy. Beware of the unexpected question like: "Should I divorce her?" Always be non-committal. Being a hypnotherapist does not qualify you as a counsellor, advisor or adjudicator, nor do you want to spend time as a witness in divorce hearings. Tell them, should they seek such advice, that it is not for the therapist to advise or to judge, and that your job is to help them to get better so they can make their own decision, but from a clearer mind.

Clients will often say: "I know I'm being silly" or "I know you'll think I'm being stupid" or "I know you think I've only myself to blame". What they are really saying is, please reassure me, please tell me you don't think I'm being silly. Respond to their need and reassure them. I often do this by saying that I certainly do not think they are being silly but that they are being a bit hard on themselves, considering what they have been through. Keep in mind too, the unsympathetic conditions they will often have had to live with. This is their chance to be taken seriously, so give them their full opportunity to freely make the most of being with you. A sentence often occurring in the thank you letters I receive, is along the lines of: "Throughout our sessions you never once judged me, you just listened with a caring and considerate manner". Having completed the first session, de-induce hypnosis, following some gentle words of encouragement, especially praise if they have done well.

Note: Many therapists, particularly those who have a low success rate, frown on giving any such praise or saying anything that might suggest good progress, for fear of it being thrown back in their faces by the clients who eventually fail to improve. Using the methods set out, carrying them out enthusiastically, confidently and conscientiously there need be no restricting fear of encouragement, for in those few cases of failure, the client will know that you have really tried anyway. In the thousands of clients that have sought my help with analysis, not one has ever written to complain. I wonder how many hypnotherapists, running a busy practice, can also genuinely claim that?

Sessions Two, Three and Four

One of the many benefits of using the strobe lamp to induce hypnosis is that during the ten minutes exposure, interesting case histories can be given. Not only does this occupy some of the time whilst hypnosis is induced, but here is another professional secret underlying my success, and the one referred to earlier in the note on case histories.

By relating them in the right way, enormously powerful auto-suggestions are given, though the client doesn't need to realise it. Although, as previously mentioned, one intelligent client stunned by his recovery, and despite his almost total scepticism of a successful outcome, had analysed the therapy in depth. He then realised, in his case at least, the case histories must have inspired his subconscious to change despite his intellectual rejections. "Brilliantly clever of you", he said, "you completely circumnavigated my scepticism, and it only came to me today as I puzzled and puzzled over how you could possible have cured me".

Any competent hypnotherapist will have a continuous throughput of successful and interesting cases. Please ignore any current doubts in your mind, that you could do the same for your client's because you can. To begin with you could always use those in this book, should you be starting out. So far, several cases have been mentioned and used as examples. Now pause for thought, what effect did they have on you? Did you find them informative, interesting or above all else encouraging that such results could be achieved? I hope you found all three reactions and the same reactions can be expected in your clients. But the client is receiving the information from the cases as he drifts into hypnosis, so they are more readily picked up by his subconscious. The reaction there is: "So that's how it goes, that's interesting, if that wonderful outcome could happen to him, it could happen for me and I want it to, for this seems the result to be expected". Such cases, especially in the early sessions do have powerful motivating consequences. In relating case histories, no risk should be taken of confidentiality being breached, neither should any indication that the therapist is boasting of his achievement be given, nor should in depth complicated details be gone into. Look at the samples given for a guide.

Get someone to time you reading them, and you will find they take little time to relate. A further valuable feature of relating case histories is, that you are subtly preparing him to understand the type of thing that he might find in his mind, thereby helping him to prepare for it in a way that reduces his fears. Furthermore, should a case you relate come near to some experience that has caused his repression and symptoms you will, even if inadvertently, have made the release much easier.

Sessions two, three and four are in principle, really just the continuation of the process of free association begun in the first session. But there are one or two points worth noting. Although the second session can occur even on the following day, subsequent sessions should be not less than five days apart and any gap of more than two weeks should be avoided. The 'same time next week' idea is best. This time spacing rule applies throughout the treatment with one exception. Having completed the eight-session course, a client may feel that he still needs more treatment when you feel he does not. In such a case, an appointment - the ninth, should be booked for a month ahead. This calls for some explanation.

As in any medical procedure, where a patient may be either suffering the after effects of his treatment or simply needs some opportunity to recuperate the same need can, on some occasions occur following hypnotherapy. Take the case of an appendectomy: having the appendix removed in appendicitis. Following a successful operation, the patient will feel sore and be initially partially disabled, if in response his surgeon was to take him back to the theatre for a further exploratory operation, then recovery would be delayed. No, in such a case the complete recovery needs a little time, and the patient needs to be left to recover. As the therapist, you will gain respect for yourself from the client for being honest and professional enough to give proper advice, and not be tempted to take fees under false pretenses. After all, the client can still call you sooner if he really needs you.

Where a client has gone through his therapy in a spirit of co-operation, but feels that he is still not 'quite right', this four-week delayed appointment will in most cases, bring the full cure while he waits for the next visit. Deferring that next session can be a difficult matter to judge because sometimes a ninth, tenth or more appointments will be needed and best be carried out without undue delay, but these are rare. A competent and experienced therapist, adopting the methods set out here, will mostly only need eight sessions. A typical exception would be a client having had his eight sessions requiring to attend for say, stop smoking therapy.

Another consideration of importance during the first four sessions is, that some change in the client can mostly be expected. Imagine a graph. On the left at the bottom, we have 'B' for 'feeling bad', above it at the top of the vertical left line, we have 'G' for 'feeling good', with eight equal spaces between them. On the right of the graph we have another vertical line, with our 'B' at the bottom and the 'G' at the top. If we were to plot our client's progress, week by week, like some temperature chart in a hospital, we would be amazed to see how each client's chart or graph would differ. Assuming we place him exactly half-way up on the left-hand side, he might produce a horizontal line between any sessions, even for the first seven. Alternatively he might make rapid progress to any point, heading higher up to the 'G' level, or he may suddenly start heading down towards the 'B' level, or go up one week and down the next. Alternatively, his graph may take the appearance of continuous improvement, step-by-step, week-by-week, only either to continue like that or take a sudden drop before rising again to finish at the 'G' level.

The explanation for all this is rather simple. In the course of the work you may initially remove the accumulated pressures - rather like removing the pus from an infected splinter - where the pain is lessened by the removing of the pressure. Sooner or later, like subsequently having to extract the splinter, the suffering may again temporarily return as the causal repression comes nearer to release. Of course, the client hasn't had puss but the accumulated consequences of his condition released. The release of the repression is a subsequent and different matter. Again, if the fundamental problem is, as it often is, one of the complexes, then that will not be dealt with until session six and consequently any symptoms of it will remain until then, he may be fixed at his starting point.

Alternatively, if he has say, the Oedipus Complex and quite unknown to him, and another condition that he does know about, and it is this that he has presented himself for treatment for, he may make good progress until the complex is routinely dealt with, and then have a downturn. However for most, particularly when clients start out nearer the 'G' point, sooner or later they are going to report having had a bad week, perhaps fearful that all the progress they thought they had made up until then, had been an illusion. Following a 'down' week, they may feel that their hopes are shattered and become convinced they will never recover, whereas unknown to them their set-back or bad week, is an excellent sign of progress, though they are not likely to see it that way. In more cases than not around session four, five or six, hope is at risk of abandonment by the client.

Although the client is too nice to say so, somewhere around the middle of his treatment sessions he will begin to think that the treatment isn't going to work for him; that he has not been hypnotised, or at least not in the way he expected it; that he cannot see the connection between his treatment and his problem; that everything he has told you, he knew about already; and that perhaps he's just not very good at it, or not responding somehow. The good therapist will not only watch for the signs of all this but if the signs do not show, will take the bull by the horns and bring the matter up and tell him how most people are feeling about now, mentioning the points above. If this is not done, do not be surprised if your client fails to appear around session five, or six. Especially should he begin to feel worse, as his repression begins to surface. Should he terminate his treatment he will have abandoned his attempt, abandoned you, and remain stuck with his problem, possibly in a worse form. In short, he hasn't failed you, you will have failed him.

Session Five

In every session following the first, it is a sound practice to ask the client how they were feeling during the previous week. Not only is this a courteous practice but it keeps the therapist in touch with progress. Normally the client will reply in his social habit, by saying he is "Fine", or the week has been "All right", adding "Thank you". This type of social response is not enough, the question is a medical one, and some further details are required. In particular, it helps in dealing with the points raised earlier, when the client might terminate his treatment prematurely by thinking the sessions are failing. By session five, an indepth assessment of progress before commencing therapy, is essential for additional reasons. In session five you are to report the progress or lack of it, back to his subconscious as an important part of the work. After inducing hypnosis I say that since nineteen out of twenty clients will require eight sessions, I regard the fifth session rather as the beginning of the second-half of the treatment and as such, feel it is a good time to review progress. By now I have a good understanding of him; he is feeling easy with me and has accepted me. Having told him of my intention to sum up our progress I go through and emphasise, all the good points. For example, I may proceed as follows:

"In summing up my feelings as regards progress, I would like to make a few points, I can't put them in any order of importance, so I will just raise them as they come to mind. Firstly, however, there is one point that I would like to put on top of the list though. You know, when someone comes in here and asks me to help them with some important or vital aspect of their life, I feel tremendously flattered and I thank you for that flattery. You see, I'm not just being asked to supply a loaf of bread or produce something that will wear out. What I'm being asked to do is to change a person's whole quality of life not just temporarily, but forever. It's a vitally important job and, as I say, thank you for flattering me by asking me to do it. Secondly, I have asked you to work with me in a way that for many doesn't seem a likely route to success even though it is.

However, you've got on with it,and not just that but you've done well and given me the sort of effort I need, for my work, and in quality too. Again, you've been interesting to work with, I have enjoyed your company and looked forward to seeing you each time. I respect your values, you've got a nice character. In short, I think you are what I choose to call a goodly human being! Also, in this I see myself working for your children, wife, parents, and all the others in your life, for your friends and the people who work with you, because all of us are made that bit happier by coming into

128

contact with someone who is confidently just getting on with life - just as we are that bit cast down when we come across someone down on his luck, or out of sorts. It's like dropping a stone in a pool, the ripples from our work spread out to the benefit of all. I have plenty of motivation to help you, the cause is wholly worthwhile and I thank you for that too".

Note: Whatever you do say, has to be genuine and from the heart for if it is not, the client will detect the insincerity. It may seem gushing or over the top, but if what you say is true the client will be flattered. On occasions he may even burst into tears, replying that nobody has ever spoken so nicely to him before.

In what follows next, good judgement is required. You are going to continue with a firmness, directly related to what the client can be expected to accept without feeling overtaxed or driven too hard. With the psychologically frail or badly hurt client, you will be very gentle but with those of a much harder mental make-up you will need to be more forceful, raising your voice and possibly emphasising your points in some way. In the illustration that follows, I present the more emphatic approach, following limited progress.

Having given my praise, I deliberately pause to enable him to respond or momentarily to take in what has just been said. If he does respond - his modesty will mostly restrict him - I curtail his response by what I say next. I continue: "However, there is another point I must add, a point that's far from as attractive as what I have just said. For there is something here that is far from satisfactory, something that must be faced too!" Slightly pause for a response which, if any, must be curtailed. Continuing I go on to say: "While you have been getting on with your work, while you've been doing all those things that I have just thanked and praised you for I have to tell you, your subconscious has not been keeping pace with your efforts. It's been letting you down, for you do still have your

129

problem, don't you?" I await confirmation but curtail any response, then continue: "I say that your subconscious is hiding a very guilty secret and I will justify that statement, because it has to be a secret of your subconscious as you don't know what it is that is upsetting your mind and causing the problem, do you?" (Response - and curtailed again)

"Right! I say guilty secret because that secret is upsetting you with the symptom - that must be true as well, mustn't it?" (Any response again curtailed) "You see, you don't get upset with having a secret of what you're going to give someone for Christmas, so your subconscious must have a guilty secret and that statement must be true too! I say the time has come for a vital decision to be made, and in here today! I did say, didn't I, that I was flattered to be asked to help, and as such, I don't like your subconscious failing you and hindering me. I have no axe to grind with you, but your subconscious has not yet played its full part in helping you by resolving your problem, by letting you know what its secret is. That's a failure of its duties to you, your subconscious should be co-operating with you - helping you to feel far better. Now, I am going to ask your subconscious four questions, you don't have to answer them, but if you do choose to answer, let me add this too. I shall hold you to any response you make, there will be no going back on your word, changing your stance or failing in your commitment to the answers you give".

"Before I continue, do you understand the premise upon which I shall ask the questions?" (Yes!) Good! Mind you, if your answers are negative or don't come, then I shall end our work for it is not my job to twist your arm behind your back or take some jemmy to your mind. And subconscious, can I point out to you., that if you do not co-operate, you will take (*client's name*) away today to do the best you can, and can I remind you, your best hasn't done (*client's name*) much good lately".

"Okay, here's the first question. I say that there are two parts to your life, there's the past and for all of your experiences, good bad and indifferent, the past is over and gone. On the other hand, there's your 'here-and-now' and the future and you have to live through that. You can anticipate it, mould it, enjoy it and make the most of it. Now, I say that your the subconscious should be concerning itself with perfecting the future and making the most of it rather than being more concerned with the past. (*client's name*) Do you agree that your future is the most important part of your life now, and the part your subconscious should be concerned with and concentrating its attention on? (Yes!) Good! So you choose to answer the questions, and of course, you are right. Let me emphasise the validity of your answer. I know of two psychotic patients, let's call them X and Y, who both do the same thing, for most of the day they sit on the floor, wrap their arms around their knees and bury their faces between their wrists. They will briefly acknowledge visitors, or stop to eat, or go to the toilet, but other than that, that's how they spend their days. What's happening of course is that they have withdrawn, magnetised by some past events in their lives. I can't help them but it does show how serious it can be to concentrate only upon the past. For them, there is no here and now, nor any future!"

"Right, then would you also agree, that if it is some past event that produced your guilty secret, and one that undermines your prospects for the future, that that matter should be brought to the surface, dealt with, and got out of the way? (Yes!) Good. Do you know how they produce a cultured pearl? Let me tell you. A grain of sand is inserted into the oyster, the oyster then proceeds, not to eject it, but to cover it up and hide it with a mucus which we call pearl. Of course, it then becomes a greater problem because it has been enlarged. So, the oyster follows the same procedure as before but as it does so the problem doesn't get resolved, but just keeps on getting bigger. Until eventually, the problem becomes so enlarged by the attempted faulty solution, that the oyster endures constant agony. Without going into the why of its reaction it does demonstrate the folly of attempting to conceal a problem. What the oyster should have done of course, was to have ejected that sand particle in the first place. Okay, so you agree that your future is more important to you than the past and that any guilty secret from your past should be brought to the surface and be dealt with".(Yes!)

"Good! But, as valid as those two decisions are, lets just move them to one side for a moment, as if they count for nothing, and in their place take up another issue for consideration, all by itself. I have, or have had people come in here with the most ghastly range of medical and psychological conditions and I have found that in the vast majority of cases, their conditions, are rooted in some guilty secret hidden in their minds. If for no other reason than to contribute to a longer, healthier, fitter life, would that be a good enough reason even on its own, for resolving your guilty secret? (Yes!) Good. Then here is my fourth question, will you do just that?" (Yes!)

(*Pause.*) (*client's name*) "I did say how much this work means to me as well as to you, didn't I? (Yes!) Then you will understand that I can't take any chances. You see, I think your subconscious has held its guilty secret for years, and probably even longer than you've been aware of it. Yet your subconscious appears to have done nothing about resolving it, but in here, your subconscious only having known me for about five hours, appears to have made a great decision for change. Can you understand that I might be a bit suspicious of the validity of your stated intention? (Yes!) Well I'm going to check that answer and right now".

I then move to the client's side and say: "I'm going to touch your right index finger. (*touch*) If your subconscious means what I have heard you say, that it too has had enough, and sees all the benefits of resolving it's guilty secret, by letting you know what it is, then I want your subconscious to demonstrate that commitment by causing your right index finger to react by moving now!" (Await the signal, and request it again if necessary. Ignore any movement that the client admits he has deliberately made.) The signal must be watched for carefully, because it might well be just a small nerve reaction, and may not be repeated if it is missed. Where no signal is detected, the client should be asked if he felt one or how his hand feels. Often the client, under these circumstances, will report that he did feel it or report that his hand or finger feels strange, tingling or gently throbbing. Such reports indicate the intention of the subconscious to respond with 'yes'. Should no reaction appear or be felt by the client, then the hand-holding technique should be employed. In the extremely unlikely situation where no such confirmation signal is transmitted, further negotiation with the subconscious is called for, especially to explore the possibility of some concealed motive. Personally, I have never experienced a situation where the subconscious has continued to refuse to confirm its commitment, because that would have to be illogical. However, confronted with such a unique outcome, I would press on, hoping for the best, relying on the logic of what is to follow to override the subconscious's reluctance. However, all having gone well so far as it usually does, with an open expression of pleasure I thank the client's subconscious.

An Alternative Opening Approach to Session Five

An alternative to the approach given above, is used where it is judged appropriate either because the client is still too psychologically frail or has already made significant progress. The praise is still given however, but followed by presenting the questions in a helpful, understanding caring way of reasoning, stressing more the simple logic of the benefits of change.

Where the client has already made significant progress, the questions are put forward more in the way of supporting continuing change, incorporating such statements as: "As you have already found out, such changes are welcome and beneficial", or "Your subconscious has already realised", or "Your subconscious has already commenced the process of change", or "Changes for the better are now coming faster and faster", and the like. In a few cases, it can be beneficial to allow the first part of this session to be used as an extension to the free association sessions. Whichever approach is to be made, as stressed earlier, a considerable amount of accurate judgement by the therapist is called for in deciding the best one.

Summing Up

In whatever form it takes, what is the reason for conducting the first part of session five in the manner suggested? There are two reasons.

The first is the benefit to the client, because the client's subconscious has been aware of its problem for some time, probably years, and has not only become used to having it but by now considers it a normal state. However, the procedure has now focused the subconscious's attention on it in a new way, and the importance of resolving it has been stressed, accepted and all this with the subject in hypnosis, which is in itself a totally different state of mind to the one in which he has previously only consciously wished his problem would go away.

The benefit is further enhanced because by this session, his subconscious has accepted the therapist, it has been exercised and it has become more aware of the root cause of the problem anyway. The second benefit is for the therapist for he is now going to be working on the basis that 'planning permission' for change has been given, and the need for it agreed. The therapist now has an enormously powerful argument, based upon logic and agreement that he can use, should difficulties or resistance emerge later.

For instance, should the subconscious, not wishing to 'hurt' the client's conscious mind by releasing the cause of the problem to it, the therapist can remind it that it has agreed to release him and confirmed its intention of doing so.

Quite often in session seven, this powerful argument is used and where it is it is often the crucial point that finally releases the repression.

Part Two of Session Five
The Wise Old Man

Following the successful conclusion to the first part of this session, I invite the subconscious to begin (or continue to) the release of the problem(s) by using the exercise to follow.

Sitting back behind my desk, I continue: "Now I want you to build a picture in your mind, I want you to imagine that you are going on a trip to meet a very wise old man, who lives in a cave on a mountain. You have started your journey and at the moment, have paused on the mountain track, from where you are the track slopes gently upwards. It is midnight, but above there is the biggest and brightest moon that you have ever seen. There's no movement in the air but the temperature is perfect. Wafting up from the valley below is the wonderful aroma of the pine trees, blending with the scent of the wild mountain flowers on the slopes. Say 'yes' when you are there in the picture. (Yes!) Good. Now I want you to begin moving forward, but as you go look for two large boulders, between which a soft green grass path leads off to one side, turn onto the path and say 'yes' when you have. (Yes!) Good, feel the soft grass underfoot, see the mountain flowers in it, their colours, like the grass, all changed by the light from the moon. Gone are the pinks, reds and yellows, now the flowers are white, grey and black, and the grass is a deep olive. Shortly, ahead of you among the few trees there are on this part of the mountain, you will see the occasional flicker of flame that comes from the dying embers of the wise old man's camp fire of the day. Say 'yes' when you see them. (Yes!) Good.

"The grass path curves and leads down a shallow slope and out into a small clearing. Over there is the wise old man's camp fire. See the orange red glow of the burning timbers, the brilliant white of the ash,and see too that thin strand of white smoke gently rising into the air (*pause*) and there beside the fire, is a pile of logs and over there is the entrance to the cave itself. Now go forward and pick up four or five of the logs, and drop them into the fire so that the fire crackles and flares up - and so brightly that, by the light of those dancing flames you can see inside the cave itself. Tell me what it looks like in there? (*response*) Good. Now shortly, coming towards you from the back of the cave, the wise old man will move forward to greet you. As he comes forward, describe him for me what does he wear, what's on his feet, does he have a beard?" (*client describes*) "Now, as he greets you I'm going to ask him some questions. He may answer in many ways he may smile, shrug his shoulders make some gesture with his hands, nod or shake his head, wink or say something. "What I want you to do is to tell me what he means by his reactions". I then proceed with the questions.

"Wise old man, is it possible, unlike Mr X and Mr Y, that I

mentioned earlier, for (*client's name*) to be released from his problem?" Expect 'Yes' but if 'No' (*rare indeed*) the present wise old man is a fraudster, and should be sent back to be replaced by the genuine one, and the question repeated.) "Then, wise old man, since it is possible for (*client's name*) to be freed from his condition, would you agree to use all your wisdom and efforts to help (*client's name*) do so? (Yes!) Good. Then, wise old man, with all my experience and knowledge helping him, will (*client's name*) get better? (Yes!) Good. Wise old man, (*client's name*) may need you and your help at any time in the future, to inspire him, to help him with important decisions and the like. If (*client's name*) finds that he needs that help, would you come forward and give it? (Yes!) Good.

Suddenly there is a 'crack' from the fire causing you to look at it. You see a small jet of violet-blue flame quietly hissing from a timber, tell me when you see it? (Yes!) See how beautiful it looks but now as you return your gaze to the wise old man, you see him offering you a present - what is he giving you? (*response*). The time has come for you to leave, I want you to say your farewell, and go back along the grass path, stop when you emerge from between the two boulders and say 'here' when you have. (Here!) Good".

I then discuss the present the wise old man has given. Mostly it will be symbolic but it will always have a positive meaning. A book say, either with instructions for a better life or empty, to symbolise the coming freedom to rewrite his life. It may be a diamond or some gold bar to represent goodwill and fortune in some way; a torch to help light up life in future, or a walking stick to help him on his passage ahead; a parcel either empty, signifying his problems are to be gone, or the parcel might contain something, perhaps some mess, representing his problems as being passed to him, for him to throw away or dispose of. There are countless variations but in each a positive connection exists and should be looked for.

For example, I once had a lady client who suffered with melonconic depression for many years and during session two, she told me that the only time she could remember being free of it was for about half-an-hour when she had taken her parents to the seaside. She also told me how wonderful she felt in that brief interval. When it was suggested that the wise old man was offering her a present and I asked her what it was, she responded with a protracted silence: "What is it?" I enquired, "what has he offered you?" "I don't understand", she replied, "he's given me a beautiful sea shell". (*Symbolic of course, of once again returning to feelings she had briefly experienced on the beach, and an excellent example of the subconscious's memory and pictorial thinking*).

Next, following a short discussion of the present, I ask who the wise old man is? Many will answer, 'Jesus' or 'Merlin' their grandfather and so on, but sometimes they will guess the truth, that he is their subconscious. The wise old man exercise is the bringing into contact, without the client consciously realising it, of both the conscious and subconscious minds using the subconscious's natural interpretation methods.

In conclusion, in three separate ways, four if the hand-holding technique has been applied, he has said 'yes' to his willingness to resolve his problems. The purpose in both parts of session five has been to significantly exercise his mind and concentrate it on bringing about change. Of course, he has also been prompted by previous case histories illustrating the benefits of doing so. Significant subconscious activity can now be expected in the client. During the coming week he may well hit a 'bad-patch' as the root cause of his problem does begin to surface.

Session Six

Of course, upon his arrival you ask him what sort of week he had and has he been dreaming much? This above all weeks is likely to produce reports of a down-week, if he does report a poor week of course progress is well under way. Session six is to be a packed session and I shall want to see him on his own, if possible , should he normally be accompanied, at least for the first part of the session. In this, I shall cover the appropriate complex that is either the Oedipus or Electra version. I begin by sometimes explaining a symptom can arise, not from some consciously experienced event, that is subsequently repressed and thereby hidden, but from a subconsciously produced experience, i.e., one that has its origins in the subconscious mind itself and when this has happened, it calls for a special approach, resolving the matter not through a conscious mind release but rather by dealing with it where it is. To do this I explain to the client, I must take the matter up in a way that the subconscious can easily understand, and to make sure of success I must put the issue forward in two separate ways.

I continue by saying: "What I am going to deal with soon, I go through with every client. In doing so with you, I have no way of knowing if it is relevant or not". I point out that I shall not ask them to consciously accept it as relevant, but I do ask them to agree to keep an open mind. (Although the complexes have been covered previously, in what is to follow is the suggested method of conveying an explanation to the client, and as such is different.) To simplify the procedure I adopt, the method is given divided into parts.

Note: Parts one, two, three and four that follow must be interpreted by the therapist in accordance with the therapist's personality and in a way acceptable to the client. No absolute script can be given that would always suit everybody. It is more essential that the therapist understands the principle involved than attempt to read out or memorise some script. In this way the issues can be adapted to the needs they are intended to serve. From time-to-time during the presentation, it is also advisable to check with the client as to how they are reacting, such as asking the client if they are following what's being said, or asking them to come in with any point they wish to raise, this will help keep the therapist in touch with the client's reactions.

In my years in practice, whilst the complexes have on occasion been rejected they seldom are, and I have never had to terminate my presentation of them. In response to what little negative reaction does come from the client you have those statements you made before you began. You are presenting them with an opportunity of releasing a subconscious anxiety that could possibly, have the most serious physiological as well as psychological consequences eventually, in addition to any symptom currently being suffered.

Part One
Preparation

I ask them if they were aware that a newly-born male can experience an erection when less than an hour old? This, I continue, proves three things. One, that sex is present from the very beginning, and since the sexual intensity is equal in both males and females, the same can happen to the female infant, but would be less visible of course. Two, that sex is under the control of the subconscious, since while the intelligent conscious mind exists it knows nothing at such an early stage. Three, the reaction of the erection shows that the subconscious lacks intelligence for if it had any it would realise the reaction is fruitless. The reaction itself stems from the desire to copulate and is a response to the preservation of the species reflex action, arising from the fear induced by the birth itself.

Part Two
Explanation to Male Client

Now let's look at what's going to happen to the male infant. Over the first months and years, his mother is going to love him, wash him, bathe him, dress him, tickle him, take him out, sing to him, talk to him, play with him, feed him, etc. etc. In all of this of course, his mother is female and he is male. What is he going to make of all this attention? Her beautiful looks, wonderful aroma, kindness, soft touch and understanding? Why, that a special and highly attractive relationship exists between them and of course, all this with sexual overtones too and with the intelligent conscious mind making little contribution, his subconscious is going to start arriving at its own conclusions and ideas. Namely, that his mother is his partner but bigger, more authoritative and cleverer than him, and that the gap must be closed. He must grow up and be seen as successful and more equal. He is subconsciously sexually in love with her, having an affair if you like.

Sooner or later however, he is going to become aware of rivals, in the form of sisters or brothers perhaps. However, there is one major rival he becomes aware of, his father. Gradually he becomes more and more aware of the father, subconsciously resenting him and the advantages he has over him. He may become subconsciously fearful of being found out by his father, and his subconscious might well reflect this in his dreams, where he pictures himself pursued or threatened. Indeed, his perception of being threatened may be more real than it is imagined for his father may well, even if much later, subconsciously pick up the signals being transmitted by the son to his mother particularly if, as they often are, similar signals are transmitted back from mother to son.

It must be emphasised, not only are both mother and son intellectually ignorant of what is going on, being left only with subconscious inclinations and feeling towards each other, but that each would strenuously deny any such allegation, especially in maturity. However sooner or later, perhaps when he is packed off to school as if no longer needed at home, the son will perceive his battle as lost, although the subconscious programme is never cancelled, but just left as it is with any of the thousands of possible permutations that may have resulted. Those early emotions and experiences remaining locked into his mind, will have changed him, and effect him for the rest of his life in many ways. This programming may remain undetected even forever, or suddenly spring into effect in some way, with some experience or event yet to come.

Following my explanation, I tell my client that what I have just described is called the Oedipus Complex and then, much as if some afterthought, or in some casual sense of interest, ask: "Do you think it may, in some way, have played a part in your life too?". Where the response is one of doubt, I leave it at that because his subconscious will know the truth, and in bringing the mature intellectual reasoning and rational explanation to bear, the task of removing the effects of the complex are achieved in any case. Where the client is gifted with greater insight, and especially where the complex can more readily be seen as the cause of some important negative aspect of his life, I often discuss the subject in a way more relevant to his case and his experiences, before going on to the next part of the session.

Part Three
Explanation to the Female Client

The female, following her birth, will be looked after by her mother who will of course, do everything for her. Showing her love, attention and kindness, she will dress, bathe, wash, kiss, tickle, talk to and sing to her. She will put her to bed, be with her when she awakes and comes when she cries out. During all this her sexuality will come into action from time to time, who is there but her mother to point it at, and be the object of it but her mother? But somehow it doesn't quite fit, there's something missing, the sexual aspect is not completely fulfilling, it's as if she needed something else. The intelligent mind is of little help, the subconscious must make the most of the situation, while lacking the intelligence necessary to get things into perspective and draw accurate conclusions. The programme of attachment is laid down; she must close the gap between her and her mature, intelligent, authoritative mother, to secure the relationship in the satisfying way it is currently felt and enjoyed.

As the weeks and months pass, she is to become aware of another figure in her life. That figure is a man (brother, uncle, grandfather or other) but most likely her father. He is different to her mother, slightly dangerous in a sense, but also a little mysterious, exciting and intriguing. All these reactions are going to incline her sexuality towards him. Leaving her with a subconscious dilemma of choice between father and mother. A fascinating attraction to her father develops, that conflicts with the security she needs from her mother. She needs both, but feels that she must choose between them.

Her subconscious is going to express her plight in its dreams; what if she were to be found out as it were, and then goes on to project this fear of discovery, by seeing herself pursued. She may be pursued in her dreams by a witch or monster yet never caught, because she never is found out in the way she fears, but in another way, because she cannot help herself transmitting her signals of infatuation and especially where these are returned, they will be intercepted by the mother. Without realising it consciously, the mother may now develop an attitude of jealousy or enmity towards her daughter later in life. As an alternative response or perhaps in addition, the daughter having lost the competition with mother for father's attention she may be inspired by jealousy herself. However subconsciously, the infant female may instead perceive the switch of her love from mother to father as if an act of disloyalty. As a result, a further conflict may arise, because the infant girl now wants to do everything she can, to retain and secure her original relationship with her mother.

In all of these mental conflicts and desires, little intelligence is brought to bear and subsequently her non-intelligent subconscious has to develop its own plans. She may decide on a never-ending expression of loyalty to her mother and feel guilty for selecting her father as her choice for the time she did. Earlier she had programmed herself to go on trying to make the relationship with her father complete in every way. If later, her father proves himself to have been unworthy of her intentions, she may grow to hate him, desperately seeking a replacement that will give her the satisfaction she once sought. These early conflicts may continue to effect her in her future relationships, and in many other ways too. Added to all the possible permutations of reactions, is to be added the greatest complication of all, i.e., in the way it was originally intended to develop, her relationship with her father comes to nothing. She is ultimately going to have to exchange him for another male.

Part Four
Presentational Conclusion

To be presented to clients of either sex, adjusting the male/female terms accordingly.

Continue thus: "Let's imagine you have a friend, one that

you've known for years and that you meet from time to time. One day, your friend greets you in an enthusiastic and excited manner. Your friend can't wait to tell you that they had met someone, a few weeks ago that is 'out of this world' and begin to describe him/her. Saying how they met, what they've done, what they're planning, and how truly wonderful he/she is, and how excited he/she feels. It's as if, for your friend, the world has suddenly opened up to them. Your friend is walking on air and is already deeply in love. From time to time you continue to meet your friend, always to hear the same enthusiastic subject eagerly talked of. You've never known your friend to be so happy and radiant".

"One day, almost beside himself/herself with joy, your friend approaches you and can't wait to tell you his/her great news a proposal for marriage has been made and accepted. In your friends enthusiasm you are repeatedly pressed to confirm that you will attend the wedding to which you repeatedly agree. No fixed date has actually been concluded but this will be agreed that evening, and you are assured that your invitation will be in the post, to arrive the next morning. Your friend then leaves to pass the good news to another friend. You've never known anyone so smitten by love, and you feel very happy for him/her. You are wondering just what this 'magical' prince/princess must actually be like. You can't wait to meet him/her. Now, you have your wedding present to choose, new clothes to buy, you wonder what date will have been chosen because you have a full diary yourself. Now you are caught up in this thing".

"Next morning you eagerly scan your post, but there is no invitation card amongst it. The next day's post arrives the following morning, but still no card. Day begins to follow day until a week has gone by. Still no card and you have not seen your friend either. Curious! The following week begins, and it too proceeds through its course, bringing no card or any meeting with your friend. Curiouser

145

and curiouser! Now a third week begins to run its course, still no card, still no contact with your friend".

"On the Thursday you meet a second friend, one that you also see from time to time. You explain your concern at not having seen or heard from your first friend. Your second friend responds that they are in the same position and are curious too. Your second friend tells you that the first friend usually goes to a pub called the Rose and Crown on the other side of town for a sandwich lunch on most days. And suggests that it might be a good idea for one of you to pop in to see if your mutual friend is there and to find out what's happening".

"You decide that you will go. Accordingly, the next day you arrive at the pub. It is a bright sunny day so that when you first enter your eyes take a few moments to adjust. It's quite a busy place and your initial inspection fails to detect your friend. As you begin to wonder if you should ask someone if they have any news, or knows anything, a door to a back room swings open as a customer passes through. You catch a glimpse of what might be your friend, sitting in the corner of the next room all alone and looking greatly unhappy. His/her clothes look as if they have been slept in, his/her hair is a mess and his/her shoes muddy. As you approach you wonder what to say. Fortunately you are spared your concern for your friend is anxious to meet you and to pour out his/her grief. Your friend is now in a highly emotional state and tells you that it is all over, the romance is shattered and he/she is near suicidal. You press for details. Why, what's happened? Your friend does his/her best to explain. It seems your friend's partner had never intended things should have gone as far as they did. It had been intended by the other partner to be a temporary, more casual thing but that as it unfolded, the other partner just couldn't bring himself/herself to say so".

"The time was never right, there was never an opportunity

to spare your enthusiastic friend's feelings. Somehow, it couldn't be done and the situation just snowballed and got entirely out of hand. Finally, your friend continues by saying that when the date for the wedding had to be chosen, the issue was forced to a critical point. It transpired that the partner was already married and that the spouse, who had been away, is due to return any day now. Your friend says they know the spouse and that person is a really terrible type. Your friend has told everyone of the relationship so the spouse is bound to find out and will come looking for them. So, says your friend, I have lost the greatest love I have ever known and gained a terrible enemy too. I don't know what to do or how to cope, my life is in ruins. I have made a fool of myself. Your friend then continues in the same vein".

(*client's name*) "If such a thing really happened it would indeed be a catastrophe for the victim involved wouldn't it? (*agreement*) But lets swap the victim for you. So that it's you in the chair, and begin to run time back, so that instead of you being your age now, you become twenty, fifteen, ten, nine, eight, seven, six, five or four and imagine that the principles of what happened in the story, have just happened to you!"

"Can you see what an unprecedented disaster it would be, what confusing decisions and conclusions your subconscious could arrive at? The hopelessness, anger and guilt feelings you might have? How you might - with the subconscious having a perfect memory of it for life - become depressed, angry, begin to lack confidence or subconsciously go on to feel the pain and frustration forever? And see how that could lead to disastrous consequences for some bodily part, if quite unrealised by you that part began failing under the continuing stress. Do you think that this complex might, even just might have entered your life in some way or degree too?"

In response to your question the client may react in many

ways, some will say "yes!" Some, "possibly". and a very few say "no!" - their response doesn't matter because it will come from the client's intelligent conscious mind and, in hypnosis your client's subconscious has listened and it knows the truth, and that truth is that "yes!" it did happen. But with your explanation of it, it is able to adjust and see things as they were then and how they are now for the first time.

The effect of either the Oedipus or Electra Complex on your client could have existed to any of a wide degree of depths, but it would mostly have been there, and your explanation will either have resolved it or triggered the resolution through a new understanding. Your explanation has been given and is to be found especially worthwhile in some seven cases out of ten. If your client was not significantly a victim himself, you have still given him information that could be of great value in helping him understand those around him better. If you are right, as mostly you will be, then you will have changed his life for the better and forever, although you will never know which client's they are, from time to time you will be saving their life too. I am satisfied that above all else, the two complexes are a prime causal factor that produce some unexpected heart attacks and many other serious conditions as well.Since session six is a busy one, it is necessary to curtail the discussions which the client might be tempted to engage in following the complex explanation. Such discussions will be little more than similar to symptom discussion and this takes time and achieves little. Instead, tactfully move on to the next session six exercise.

Neuro Linguistic Programming
(N.L.P.)

With some clients, N.L.P. will cause little if any significant reactions, but in many it will. In about one-in-five cases, these reaction can also be intensely emotional. N.L.P. can be compared to a directed dream experience but carried out in hypnosis rather than sleep, with the conscious mind making a significant contribution to the process. Amazing improvements can follow it, sometimes instantly too. It is particularly relevant where the client has been a significant victim of one of the complexes. It can also be useful with client's that have had a difficult childhood, a past relationship problem or in coming to terms with the loss of a deceased loved one. During the process, the subconscious is drawn to matters that concern it, and in conjunction with the conscious mind attempts to resolve them and in so doing, mostly succeeds.

To begin the process, I usually remind the client that in session five we imagined visiting the wise old man, and say that I want to go through a similar exercise again. I tell the client though that I want him to explore his own mind, and since I can't expect him to imagine himself clambering through a lot of assorted grey material, I shall ask him to imagine that his mind is made up of rooms, corridors, cupboards and the like, rather like an office. I then continue: "So to begin with, imagine yourself just standing in a lovely broad corridor, well lit and wonderfully decorated. Say 'yes' when you are there". (Yes!)

Note: Occasionally a client may have, at first, some difficulty at attempting this. If he does, encourage him and if he should find continuing difficulties it is most likely to be because the explanation of the complex is still seriously distracting his subconscious, particularly if he managed the previous visit to the wise old man easily. As such, it is a good sign that you were right in putting the concept forward. You may, in cases where the inability to imagine the scene continues, return to free association or take up some other issue, because in such cases his mind is still too busy to concentrate on imaginative things.

Assuming the client, as most do, goes along with the requested imagining by responding with that 'yes', continue: "Good, now I want you to become aware that you are standing on one of the most luxurious carpets you've ever walked on, so look down and tell me what colour or colours it is made up of?" Often he will say red, meaning that his subconscious feels anger or determination. Alternative colours can mean other feelings: brown, subconsciously feeling messy; blue, I feel good, relieved, or want to feel good; yellow, I am looking for or expecting a new beginning, a fresh start; green, I feel optimistic; grey, I am feeling neutral; purple, there is a sexual matter that bothers me; pink, I'm thinking of my mother or with the female client, perhaps, "I'm female and proud of it"; no colour can be taken as hard fact, but you will have at least a possible guide to the client's feelings.

Having received the colour answer, I then invite the client to begin to move down the corridor until he reaches a door, and that when he can see it he should again say 'yes'. (Yes!) "Good! Now through that door is a room that contains all the units which control every aspect of your body and mind. Those units may appear as computer terminals, filing cabinets, cupboards or control panels. Now I want you to enter and describe what you see". (*client describes*) "Good! Now, are there any warning lights or any other indications that show anything to be wrong?" If the client says 'No', get him to check again but do not suggest that you expected warning lights or signals.

If 'No' again, proceed with part 'B' below. If your client reports such a light, lights or signals, ask him to go over to it, or to the nearest one if there are two or more, and tell you what that unit controls or does for him. He may not know what that unit does for him but more often he will have some idea. For example, a lady client finding such a warning light said the unit looked after her hair, and commented that she had been very worried about a serious recent hair loss. She imagined herself rectifying the unit and the fault indicating light going off, when she had done so. She was to ring me, several weeks after her treatment in a state of high emotion, to say her home hairdresser had just asked her what she had used to restore her hair to such luxurious healthy growth.

Where a fault indicating light or signal is reported, next ask what is wrong with the unit. If they don't know, suggest a computer disc may be jammed; some wire could be loose; that the unit is not tuned in properly; or make similar suggestions. Encourage them to find the fault and then to remedy it in some way - even to see themselves replacing the unit if needs be. If they encounter some difficulty ask them to look for an internal telephone.

When they have found it, ask them to ring for the wise old man and tell you when he's arrived. In this approach, when your client says the wise old man is there, tell your client to indicate the problem to him and watch as he carries out the repairs until the warning light or signal goes off. Repeat similar exercises for any other fault indications, either with or without the wise old man, according to whether he has been sent for or not. This procedure, which often seems just like a game to the client, can have amazing effects for in it, you are using the natural subconscious's thinking and healing methods.

Part B

Any such fault indications having been dealt with, continue but now in an almost apprehensive or concerned sort of voice, thus: "Now, somewhere in that room is another door, not the one you came in by, but another. Say yes when you see it. (Yes!) Now in a moment, not yet, I will ask you to cross the room and go through that door, closing it behind you, and when you have, stand rigidly still with your back to the door and say yes when you are there. Please do

151

that now". (Yes!) Next continue, speaking more slowly and softly with the approach being intended to heighten the intensity and expectation of the client. Look slowly around the room and tell me is there somebody already in there? (If No!) "Look around again, look for any shadow that might mean someone's hiding behind a pillar, curtain or cupboard". If no indication of another person initially results, persist a little longer or continue by saying: "Okay, since this is your mind, we can think of this room as your managing director's office, and in that case, there is an adjacent room to this one, that is used for people waiting to see you. Tell me when you can see the door that leads to that room". (Yes, having come this far, a No is most unlikely.) "Good, then go in there and tell me who is waiting for you".

Note: Sooner or later the client in most cases will find someone or some people. These will be those who either are or have been, important to them in some way, and most often they will fit into one of four broad categories. One, their current love, and following the complex explanation, this often signifies their freedom to love them. Two, some perpetrator of harm. Three, relatives or parents, or the parent of the opposite sex, again often a complex related imagery or four, some deceased family relative or friend. The variations, feelings, reactions and experiences are so many that only an idea of what the therapist is to have his client do can be given here. In essence the event has to be of a constructive positive nature, making up, embracing, forgiving and the like. Where the attempt to release any animosity fails, ask the client to tell the person to leave and watch him go. He should see himself tell that person to go in a controlled positive way. Commonly there will be tears of a happy, sad or angry nature.

When the exercise is completed in the managing director's office or the waiting room, ask your client to go back to his control-room and when he has arrived, to say if any new warning signal has come on while he's been busy out of the room. If 'Yes', proceed as earlier, or if 'No', as it mostly will be, ask him to return to the corridor and say 'yes' when he is there. (Yes!) "Now I want you to realise that while you have been doing your work the carpet fitters have been in and laid a brand-new carpet, look down at it, and tell me what colour or colours do you see now?"

The colours will again portray his subconscious feelings. If you have been conscientious in your work, and used an underlying tone of enthusiasm in dealing with whatever situations may have arisen, you will have brought about positive changes though you may not be able to name those changes, they are most likely to be reflected in the colour or colours to be reported to you in the new carpet. Hope above all, for yellow and more especially gold, meaning I see new opportunities and/or a fresh start, or green for optimism and blue for feeling good.

Session Seven

By this time most clients will mostly report feeling better in some way; they may even be boastful of their recent personal achievements, now being freer of their previous symptoms and possibly they may dismiss, out of hand, any interest in some previous symptom now regarding it as irrelevant. Most will have come a long way from the original starting point they presented to you on your first meeting, but expect about one-in-five to report little if any progress though. While this is naturally disappointing to both, when such negative reports are made at this stage take heart, for you have a session seven 'tool kit' that hasn't even been used yet.

Here's how to proceed. Take the client into hypnosis, and deepen this into the somnambulistic state. Get him to help you draw up a statement representing his most important outstanding

153

requirements, one that you can read back to his subconscious. An example statement might be as follows: "Subconscious, Harry reports to me that he continues to suffer agony with his migraine, and that this agony is ruining his life. Further, subconscious, Harry reports that his social life is ruined and that he can no longer concentrate on his work. Subconscious, Harry desperately needs to be released from his awful condition and asks that you release him and in here today. Subconscious, you know what it is that occurred in Harry's life and caused his migraine and his suffering, Harry wants you to return to that incident that original experience, and pass the memory of it back to him. Subconscious this is an easy and simple thing for you to do.

Focus in on that memory clearly, so when shortly I count to three and click my fingers, you do pass that memory to him. Subconscious I will read this statement to you twice more, as you get ready to do so". (*read the statement twice more*) Then say to the client: "You are going back Harry, back to a time when the event that caused your migraine actually occurred, or to a time it is just about to occur". (*Be positive and confident - this is going to happen, just as you say it will*) "One, two, three, click!". A moment's pause, then prompt with such questions as: "Are you inside or out?" "Is anyone with you?" "What's happening now?" "How do you feel?" etc. Around fifty to sixty percent of such cases will immediately produce the abreaction required, producing the sort of result given in the case histories quoted.

Often by clues being given that lead up to it. The client may report being aware of some feeling, or see something that doesn't make sense. Unless the abreaction, in mostly an emotive state, comes out in full, further prompting may be needed such as: "Okay. subconscious, I will count to three and again click my fingers and you add to that memory (or feelings) you have just had, with something else, but always coming nearer and nearer to the actual

154

moment that led to Harry's awful migraine".

If, after several attempts you have been unsuccessful, there are other tools in your session seven kit that you can then use. Don't forget the agreement reached in session five and remind his subconscious that it did agree to bring about change and that you know the agreement will be honoured. Hand-holding or negotiating can also produce excellent results, or you can use the following method:

"Subconscious, Harry desperately needs you to release him from his awful migraine and you may do so in anyway you feel most appropriate. You may release him by causing him to have some feeling, like causing him to feel he is floating, feeling as if he is spinning, being pushed back into the chair, tipping sideways or some other sensation. You may have him feeling himself going down a tunnel, and out into the light, by just throwing the emotion to the surface, giving him that memory or a thought. When I count to three and click my fingers subconscious, you carry out that release, and in any manner appropriate. One, two, three, click!"

With a little patience and using these methods in various combinations, nine out of ten clients will have responded or will have begun to. By using your initiative, you may further encourage the client, saying such things as: "It is coming through, you are getting there, your subconscious is recalling and releasing the event", etc. Don't rush your client and above all, remain positive and patient. Should you continue to experience difficulties, tell your client you are going to take another issue or symptom, should there be one, while his subconscious continues to release in this case, his migraine. There will often be something else. Where there is another symptom or issue there is no real need to write a second statement since the client's subconscious will understand the principle by then. Because of this, an unscripted repetition of an approach similar to the original one can now be expected to bring the desired result. Sometimes, a secondary issue will not only be successful in its own right but directly lead to a successful outcome of the first attempt. Conversely, having gained a first abreaction, you may well be amazed at the simple ease with which other issues or symptoms release themselves. With abreactions now coming one after the other until, if there are say, four or five on your list, some may even be released upon merely being mentioned. My personal record is eight in a row. Abreaction releases and memories just popping up in just a few minutes while I had spent half-an-hour releasing the first.

Following this session, often the most productive, revealing and satisfying one, expect your client to feel mentally drained. If he is, that's an excellent technical sign of good progress. Despite any doubts of success you may initially have had session seven is likely to demonstrate most effectively the enormous healing powers of hypnotherapy, to your client, any attending guest and not least, to yourself, a magnificently satisfying experience to all.In this series of books, only a tiny fraction of my experiences have been illustrated and some, with a great feeling of immense personal satisfaction, will live with me forever, and, what I have done starting from scratch, you can do too, while enjoying your experiences with equal satisfaction as well.

The Solution of a 32-Year-old Mystery

During the latter stages of an analysis - especially where the first four sessions of free association have 'exercised' the mind well - amazing revelations can surface. Just such an example was to occur with a mother and her 31-year-old daughter.

In the seventh visit of the daughter, following the one, two, three, click procedure, she began to cry so intensively that I thought to fetch her mother, who was waiting for her seventh session downstairs. Initially, all my encouragement and efforts failed to break into her grief and to get her to respond to my urgent enquiries as to what was upsetting her so much. Eventually she cried out: "Don't leave me - don't go!" Reassuringly I told her I had no intention of leaving her. In due time she responded to me: "Not you - my twin sister". Intensely curious, since there had been no previous mention of a twin sister, I went over to my desk to check her notes. No indication of there ever having been a twin was to be found. Clearly some tragic experience of loss, perhaps in a previous life was being encountered.

I returned to her side and as sympathetically and cautiously as I could, pointed out that there was no reference to her twin in my notes and I asked her to give me more details of what she meant. She then went on to explain that she had found herself back in her mother's womb with her twin sister, at three months into gestation. She had become aware that her twin was 'slipping' away and had become highly emotional. Eventually, although she had been highly distressed, she regained her composure and left.

Some might justifiably say that this was just her imagination, or some horrible 'trick' of her mind except for what was to be revealed by the mother on her last visit to me the following week. She told me that her daughter had related her experience and said this had solved her 32-year-old mystery. When she had been three months pregnant with her daughter, she suffered a serious haemorrhage. The doctor had been called to the emergency and told her how sorry he was to inform her she had miscarried. Following the medical attention she still felt that 'something' was not as it should have been.

Further tests and consultations resulted. Finally, she was confronted by her baffled doctor who said he couldn't explain what had happened, but he was now very pleased to confirm that she had not lost her baby but was in fact still pregnant. Whilst personally I hold no strong feelings on the heated debate on abortion, this case has given me much food for thought.

Note: It was put forward in Chapter One that the human spirit probably takes up 'occupation' of the foetus at around five, six or seven months into gestation. But that's not to say that memories and experiences cannot be recorded prior to occupation, because in the absence of the spirit the mind within the brain continues to function fully.

Session Eight

Rather like the first session being the beginning or the opening of the case, the eighth session is rather the tidying up and closing one. It may be devoted to suggestion therapy, like smoking cessation, confidence building, or some other work may be need to be done. By now your client is mostly a million miles from where he was when he first met you. In a very small number of cases, especially where the client's symptoms have been protracted and resulted in years of suffering, such as a bad childhood, as opposed to some single event like nearly drowning on one occasion, a further session or two might be called for, especially in those very few minority cases where insufficient or only slow progress has been made. However, where the lack of progress is significantly absent a further consideration is required as to why?

When little or even no progress has been made, several possibilities present themselves. Is the client still as he is because he simply needs time for his recovery, i.e., does he need to adjust in some way? If everything has gone as it should, but the client does not yet feel completely recovered, invite him to see how he goes over the next month before consulting you again. Most such clients will never need you again or if they do, they will either consult you to merely 'tidy' them up so to speak, or they will mostly be very responsive on that next visit. Again, do they subconsciously want to get better? Sometimes their symptom can be like a cover or some protection. If this is the case, it is as if some causal accident is not resolved but continuing. The need for the symptom must be found and dealt with by negotiating, preferably using the hand-holding technique. There is also the possibility the client has been unable to broach some subject, even now, or be subconsciously hiding something from you either intentionally or unintentionally. Perhaps, although it came into his mind, a memory had occurred but had been quickly changed, rather in a fashion we experience in the: "I was going to tell you something but it's gone out of my mind". He may have thought of some subject and considered it as being of no importance, or thought he had brought it up previously. Conversely, he may have done so but in only an incidental way. Again the client may have dismissed some revelation as silly and subsequently kept it to himself. The unresolved issue has to be probed for and dealt with before relief can finally be achieved.

Another problem which can occur, although very very rare with these techniques, is the intrusion of the transference factor mentioned previously. The therapist is taken up by the client as if essential to his subconscious. In transference, the symptoms may need to continue to maintain the relationship and contact with the therapist, particularly with the lonely client and those in an unhappy environment. Transference will reveal itself by the clients obvious satisfaction with, or interest in, his relationship with the therapist, by treating the therapist in some special regard or transferring onto the therapist the feelings they had or should have for another. A break in the relationship, say for a month until the next appointment will mostly result in any transference dissipating itself, with the client ringing to say he no longer feels he needs that next appointment.

Inevitably in just a few cases, some clients will, for some irresolvable reason fail to release their symptom despite all efforts. In at least half of such cases the release will, subsequently, suddenly or gradually be achieved over the months ahead. However, it must be re-emphasised that complications are exceptional, rather than usual and should in no way discourage you. By following and using the analysis method set out here you will find that success is common place not unusual, and the time will soon come, if you have the little courage needed to try, when you will discover this for yourself.

In Conclusion

When I first started in practice, and as many talented people still do, I began with a correspondence course, having seen no actual analysis conducted. Using eight sessions of free association only I still enjoyed highly successful results. In this series of books you have a considerably greater range of tools at your disposal and a far greater range of knowledge than I then had. All you need to do is read the material until you understand what is intended by it, apply your imagination, sincerity, insight, patience, perseverance, inspiration and understanding and you too will enjoy the delights of amazing successes. Go to it, there is a mass of people waiting for your help. Hypnotherapy is a most rewarding and satisfying occupation, and for the clients, bringing great benefits for life.

Chapter Six

Treating Children and Further Techniques

The more established a hypnotherapist becomes the more likely he is to be called upon to treat children. These may be considered as clients twelve years of age and younger. Whilst I have successfully treated a child then aged three-and-a-half years old, generally I prefer them to be five or above. The success rate, particularly the younger a child is, can be less than that for adults, for three main reasons.

Firstly, the child is far more likely to be presented at the behest of the desperate parent and the child may have little incentive to co-operate. Secondly and lacking maturity, the child may see little reason for changing especially where his problem is anti-social behaviour. Thirdly, particularly with the six, seven or eight-year-old children, he has more often than not been trundled around several child specialists and all to no avail, for him it has become some sort of a game in which he has become the centre of attention. In the last case, he probably believes that he has more to lose by co-operating and changing than he has to gain. Generally, unsociable behaviour will be the presenting problem other likely conditions include bed-wetting, dreams, nightmares, withdrawal, jealousy of other family members, particularly younger ones, speech difficulties, stealing, lying and self-defecation.

In my experience, over eighty percent of children brought to me are boys. In those, by far the most likely problem is that, whatever the basic cause of their neurosis it has become, through their eyes, a valuable bond between them and their mother and

161

because of this they need it to continue. The mother will report her enormous concern to the therapist, often emotionally and in a pleading way while the child happily plays with some toy or seeks to interrupt the proceedings to ensure the spotlight remains on him. The mother mostly remains not only unaware of what is happening but also unaware of the fact that her often sympathetic reaction to him is actually egging him on, especially where the child is using his condition to gain attention.

The therapist should be friendly but firm, expecting the child to co-operate and with such children, generally those who perceive themselves to be the unhappy victim of their malaise, success rates are as high as those for adults. The most grateful client of all can be the caring parent of the child successfully treated.

Children less than nine years old, mostly require only two sessions. Since children, by dint of their age, cannot be far removed from the time when they had an experience that became repressed. The first session may bring only limited benefit. Where it has, it is possible that the child has not co-operated enough, misunderstood his role, had been distracted in some way or felt too self-conscious to act freely. It may have been the presence of his mother, in whose company he felt too shy to respond fully. When the child returns for his second session, say two weeks later and has noticed some improvement, he will be far more ready to co-operate enthusiastically since he now has an insight into the benefits of doing so.

Additionally, on the second visit he is returning to the more familiar rather than entering the unknown and strange. If his mother's presence is a restricting or intimidating factor the child may well indicate this on his return. If he doesn't, it does no harm to suggest to the mother that she asks the child if he would rather she stay. If the child indicates that he would prefer his mother to leave, she should do so.

162

However some other person, preferably another member of the practice should be present. No therapist should conduct treatment with those under sixteen years old while alone, and the younger the child the more this rule becomes essential. It is more particularly the case when the therapist is male. Notwithstanding this, where the person is say ten years old or more and they express a desire to be alone with me, I will concur but at least have someone sitting just outside the room.

Such precautions, especially since to the general public the 'mysterious hypnosis' is to be used, need no explanation to justify save to remind ourselves that as therapists, we are dealing with and treating the young immature human that is a child and one that is neurotic too. This is a combination best not left entirely to the therapist to manage and take exclusive responsibility for.

Children are normally far less questioning of treatment methods and are usually more curious and less distracted by other considerations than adults. As a result they can respond extremely well and in only the two sessions, to a degree that an adult would require a full eight session analysis course to achieve. So too, a child successfully treated, is going to benefit for life rather than being left, either to live with his conditions as most such people do or perhaps with luck, resolving his problem after many years of a distorted life when he is, say in his twenties or older.

Children would appear for hypnotherapy far more frequently if it was more widely known how they could often be helped and so easily. There are four principal approaches that can be expected, not only to have good results but even amazing outcomes. The four principal therapies that I use with children are: 'suggestion analysis', 'instant analysis', 'shortened analysis' and 'blow aways'.

Suggestion analysis is used where the young client is aged eight years or less and either cannot, or will not respond vocally. The intention here is to release the trapped emotion rather than discovering its cause. Normally two session are called for. Instant analysis is used where the client is between six and thirteen years of age. The intention here is to help release the client from his problem in a participatory way. Two to three sessions may be required. Shortened analysis is used in cases where the client is aged fourteen to nineteen years and consists of sessions one, two, three, five, six and seven of full analysis. Blow aways can be used with clients of any age, but in the young, those up to the age of eight or nine they have the special benefit that neither the cause of their problem nor any emotion need be revealed.

These benefits are attractive to those children wishing to keep some personal secret or merely feel they would lose face in displaying emotions. In the adult, the same principal action is taken, but in both cases it is used to resolve some aggravation that the client is consciously aware of. This method requires two sessions for the young and normally only a few minutes for the adult when conducted during analysis.The case of the youngest client I have had, so far, a three-and-a-half year old, will serve to illustrate the suggestion analysis method of treatment.

The Boy Whose Mother Brought Him a Present

His mother rang to say that her son lost his ability to talk, since he had been two-and-a-half; up until then she said, he was able to talk the same as any other child of that age. Then suddenly he had resorted to uttering only meaningless sounds. My initial reaction was that she should wait until he was at least nearly five because, not only was he so young for my normal therapy but he would also be quite unable to tell me anything that might help me. The mother pressed me, saying she spent the previous year going from one specialist to another and had as a result, several reports from specialists she thought would help me. However, on examination, all the reports only confirmed what she already knew, namely, that the boy had a speech problem and that if it continued he would require special educational facilities later when he began school. Against my better judgement, but out of sympathy for mother and son I agreed to see him wondering how I could treat him. In fact, it was to be his case that inspired the suggestion analysis approach to me.

Mother and son duly arrived and with the mother looking on, I induced hypnosis in the readily co-operative boy by using the strobe lamp. Having done that, I asked him to close his eyes and then began to suggest to him a list of things which I thought may have upset him. I had decided to take this approach since any communication was bound to be one sided and I did not want a situation to develop where he might find something that he wanted to talk to me about when, from the outset he could not and thereby run the risk of inducing a further subconscious frustration. I wanted him to think of the concepts that I was to put to him and to invite him to respond emotionally.

Talking in a suggestive and almost accusative manner, I began: "I think you have been worrying. I think you may have been frightened. Have had bad dreams. I think something has happened to cause you to stop talking. I think you may have been frightened that mummy didn't love you. Perhaps you've been angry or you thought mummy might leave you. Maybe you've been frightened by something on television. Perhaps you've been frightened by some people. Or someone special to you. Maybe you feel you've been cheated or left out. It may be that someone has hurt you or said something that upset you. I wonder, was there a time when you wanted to say something important, and the words wouldn't come. Some children can feel frightened of, say storms or dogs.

Sometimes boys feel sad, because they can't do things they see grown-ups do. Some boys might misunderstand a thing, and feel angry, frightened or hurt. I think something has happened to you that has made your words get stuck. Just think of all these things. Just keep thinking of them. While I say them all again. And, as I say them all again, you start thinking of what it was that happened, that made you stop talking normally. Think of it, remember it. Just let that time come back into your mind. You can see it now, and you see it more clearly all the time. Now, as you think I will say those things I said before, all over again".

The statements were put to him once again. During the course of the second listing he began to weep, gently at first and continued until he was clearly very upset. After a few moments, he relaxed and his mother comforted him. What little the child tried to say was no more coherent than when he arrived. His mother looked me in the eyes and in a voice filled with exasperation and tinged with anger, enquired: "Is that it?" Several possible replies came to my mind, regarding the reluctance to treat him that I had previously expressed to her and the advice I had given her to defer the attempt. Instead, I found myself saying: "Yes, please bring him back in two weeks time". Clearly unimpressed, she jerked her young son from the chair and left. I never expected to see either again. However, when I spoke to my wife later I was surprised that, notwithstanding what had transpired, she had made that second appointment. I was to await his second arrival, wondering what I might try next on his return. When they both returned, something was to happen that is burnt into my heart and will be there for ever.

The little boy walked in followed by his smiling mother. Before anything could be said the little boy ran a toy car along the edge of my desk, looked at me and said as he did so: "Look, the wheels go round." Following a tidying up session, the enthusiastic mother proclaimed that: "This is the finest value for money I have ever had". Oh! what was the cause of his problem? Well, it transpired that when his mother was due to have her second son, the boy was sent on holiday with his grandparents. One day, the grandparents told him his mother would be calling to take him back home and that she had a present for him. To the boy, a present meant a new toy.

Consequently, with that expectation and being keen to see his mother again he became very excited and couldn't wait to dash into the hallway when he heard the front door open. Seeing his mother, he had run up to her, his mother bent down, holding out her new baby, and said: "Look, I've got a present for you, you've got a baby brother". Instantly, the boy's speech faltered with this totally unexpected turn of events; he had not known what to say but wanted to say something, in his shock the words became garbled. It was only later that the mother realised her son had a speech problem and never connected it to the present (shock) she had given him.

Instant Analysis

In this method, the procedure is rather as for sessions seven and eight of analysis, i.e., in hypnosis, the young client is encouraged to talk of his problem in order to focus his subconscious attention on the matter, while leaving the time necessary to carry out the release. About halfway through the first session, begin by suggesting that he is: "Going back, going back to a time when something happens, or is just about to happen, that upset him so much that it gave him his problem".

Continue, by saying: "You are going back, back to that time, you are able to see it, feel it, remember it in all its details, and clearly, it's coming back into your mind now, you are remembering and recalling that time. I will count to three, click my fingers, and, if it's not already in your mind, you will just find it in your mind then. One, two, three, click!" Now help, assist and encourage him with a few questions: "Are you inside or outside?" "Is anyone with you?" "What do you see?" "What's happening?" "What happens next?" "How old are you?" "How do you feel?" and so on. With just a little effort and patience the abreaction will not almost always come to the surface but it will be possible to discuss the experience, a discussion which of itself extends the release.

However, on occasions the young client may temporarily be too emotionally overcome to discuss his abreaction and wish his mother's attention. So be it but don't push him too hard. Instead, be understanding, reassuring and encouraging, perhaps by saying, as he is cuddled by his mother. "He has played his part well, he said he would and he did.

Now he is going to enjoy feeling so much better, he is going to be so much happier. I have enjoyed working with him, I am so glad he came", or similar statements. This method, at a second session, one or two weeks later is used to explore further or to treat any further condition he may have.

The Grown-Ups Let My Grandfather Die!

I was telephoned by a desperate and tearful mother at eight o'clock one evening, begging me to see her 14-year-old son immediately. Although it followed a long tiring day, I yielded to her pleas because she told me her highly rebellious son had only just agreed he would see someone like me and as she added, he could soon change his mind.

Her son had been expelled from school on two previous

occasions for his bad behaviour and was recently temporarily suspended from another, pending a meeting of the authorities to discuss his future. All previous attempts to bring about change, including doctors, teachers, his caring parents, a psychiatrist and a social worker failed. With both his mother and father present I took the somewhat reluctant boy participant into hypnosis and began analysis. Over this and the sessions to follow it emerged that as a small toddler he had lived just a few doors from his grandfather. His grandfather had, as the father in the 'Ha-Ha Got You!' case, made much of him. The toddler visited the grandfather as often as he could. However, his grandfather began to become increasingly unresponsive to him through illness.

By the time the child was four, his grandfather was confined to his bed. The boy's visits rapidly became curtailed and then only when accompanied by his mother. The boy realised his grandfather was ill and became greatly saddened with the unfurling changes in their relationship. Eventually he was to see his grandfather lying in bed, desperately ill and requiring oxygen to sustain him. Shortly afterwards the grandfather died and the child's sadness turned to anger that the grown-ups had failed them both. "They could have saved him, grown-ups can do anything", so he became angry with them.

This subconscious anger persisted and developed as he grew and became reflected in his rebellious behaviour. In analysis came the release, and intellectual evaluation took place, change had to result and it did. Shortly afterwards, I was happy to receive a call from the boy's father expressing his gratitude and saying that his son had not only been accepted back at his school but was now doing very well. These last two cases of a non Oedipus origin demonstrate early programming resulting in negative consequences, but the consequences of the Oedipus and Electra complexes, are by far the more common.

Blow Aways

As suggested, this method is particularly suitable where the client is reluctant to talk, is shy, feels guilty or intimidated for some reason, but is co-operative to a point though otherwise limited in his responsiveness. Hypnosis is induced, possibly with the child on his mother's lap, for encouragement to give a sense of security or restraint. The purposes of restraint is to help prevent the child simply leaving the chair; distracting himself by excessive wriggling; or turning his head to gaze at some object in the room. In restraint, it is meant the gentle encouragement to sit relatively still and participate in the procedure. It often helps to boost the client's ego in some way like responding to him and treating him as if he were more equal to a grown-up; shaking his hand on arrival; talking to him and asking questions, rather than to his mother. The mother becomes the third person and the child is likely to attempt to justify your reaction and to show the maturity you expect of him through co-operating.

Unlike adults, who have plenty of time to come to totally erroneous conclusions about hypnosis and probably, as a result, would rather 'not touch it with a barge pole' if they had any choice the very young client has no such inhibitions. To him hypnosis is a tantalising prospect in which he can experience first hand, what he has read about in his comics, or seen on television. He is drawn to it, fascinated by the opportunity to have 'a go at it' rather as if he might have clamoured for a ride in some fairground, that his parents would be terrified of experiencing themselves.

Such an enthusiastic reaction to hypnosis, naturally leads itself to a heightened level of participation. Unfortunately the child may not have an enthusiastic attitude and be reluctant instead. In such a case, some encouragement will often bring about a completely different reaction. You may suggest the child is unhappy and that's sad and perhaps going to help him feel happier, and that's good. You might appeal to him in some way perhaps that he will impress his mother with how grown up he is by playing his role like an adult. Alternatively he might respond to an appeal to his ego, especially when you tell the young client he will be the first in his class and probably the only one in the entire school who was hypnotised; that he will be an authority; everyone else just talks about it but he knows the truth; perhaps he may want to tell his teacher, the class or his friends of his adventure. So hopefully now with an otherwise fidgety, less co-operative, secretive, shy, guilty or reluctant to talk child, hypnosis can be induced and you will be ready to start.

In the technique that follows you are again to give negative ideas and experiences. They are presented very much in line with the method illustrated in the case of the three-and-a-half-year-old boy. There is no fear that such suggestions might be implanted because they are given, not so much as the client is or has, but rather that some people do or some people have. Such suggestions only serving to remind your young client of something, if anything, from your list that might apply to him.

After about five or six suggestions you might say: "Now you don't have to tell anyone your secret, but just tell me have any of those things I have just said hurting you?" If he indicates 'yes' or if he has shown signs of being upset, continue with: "Then, with your eyes closed, I want you to pretend that all those awful things, memories and thoughts are in a big dirty soap bubble just in front of your face. Now here is what we will do in a moment I will count to three; when I say one you get ready; when I say two you take a big breath, and hold it. When I say 'three' you use that big breath to blow that dirty soap bubble, with all those nasty things in it away, so it hits the wall and breaks. Every nasty thing in it then just disappears, Okay?" (Yes!) "Good, say 'yes' again when you can

171

imagine that soap bubble with all those nasty things in it". (Yes!) "One, two, three" (emphasis on the 'three'). Allow a moment to pass (a slight pause of five to ten seconds) and continue: "Now, with your eyes still closed, can you imagine another dirty soap bubble, with nasty things in it floating down towards your face?" If 'yes', repeat the previous exercise and continue to do so. After five such blow aways, take of a least a minute's pause in order to avoid interrupting his breathing rhythm which could otherwise induce dizziness. (In an extreme case, blow aways being repeated in quick succession, could result in a momentary loss of consciousness). The process, in groups of five blow aways, should continue until the client reports no further such bubbles.

If, in response to your first five or six suggestions, no indication of a reaction or report of such a soap bubble is received continue with your suggestions until some such reaction or report occurs. If despite all your efforts no progress seems to been made, or as an alternative to your suggestions, another variation can be used. Suggest he begins to think himself of all the things he didn't like, the bad things in his life. "Just keep thinking of all those times when maybe you were unhappy or sad. Say 'yes' when you are thinking of something bad like that".

When he gives a confirmation that he does indeed have such a memory, proceed with getting him to use the blow away method, as earlier explained. Again, a tidying up session would be arranged. This method has considerable advantages with certain types since it also allows a repression release without the client having to tell or confess some important personal matter. However the therapist, not knowing what the cause of his problem has been is limited in what he could otherwise have done, that is to further release it through subsequent discussion. When this is the case the guardian must be told that during the interval between appointments the child's condition might even deteriorate and that if this happens it should certainly not put them off a return visit. Another advantage of this last technique is that several children could be treated together. One day perhaps, rather as we immunise children, say at the age of nine they will have their repressions erased too, saving countless spoiled lives in the process. Eventually, I think it will become normal practice especially as it becomes better known for its highly productive results.

The same Blow Away technique can be very useful in adult analysis too where a client attends a session and is distracted by some recent event or has some longer term memory of an experience which continues to intrude for instance. Of course, there is no change to reality, but rather a change of attitude towards it. The object being one of reducing or eliminating the distraction of the subject. For the adult, the technique is varied and the client is, instead of using the soap bubble instructed with his eyes closed and of course in the hypnotic state to bring up a mental picture that depicts the intruding subject and then in his own time, to take a deep breath and use it to blow the subject away visualising its disappearance as he does so. On occasions, several blow aways may be needed, perhaps with different aspects of the same subject being used.

The method has succeeded when the client can then picture the subject with a sense of detachment, reduced concern or not be able to picture it at all. I quote two examples.

It's a Green Field Now

A client stated upon his arrival for a Friday evening visit that he doubted the session would be much good because there had been a major row at work that afternoon with his boss saying it would all have to be sorted out first thing on the following Monday morning.

He said he was worried and unable to concentrate. The Blow Away procedure was explained to him, along with the suggestion that he might imagine being back in that room where the row had occurred, and the see himself blowing away his boss, or even the office he was to be in on Monday.

After several self-paced blowing aways, he was asked, since he was then smiling, just what he had blown away. "Well", he said, "I did all you suggested and then thought of the factory and blew that away too it's just a green field now".

The session was to continue productively and on his subsequent session he reported the whole matter had come to nothing anyway and he was most grateful to have been spared a weekend of unnecessary worry.

Caught Peeing in the Vicar's Garden

In the second example, a male client reported an embarrassing experience he had of being caught as a boy, by a visiting lady parishioner, relieving himself in the vicar's garden. He said that experience would often just pop back into his mind even when a remotely connected matter was experienced. Using the technique he blew away the unfortunate lady, the boy and finally, the garden. Three weeks later, he reported he had no further recurring experiences.

Re-framing

In this technique and more commonly used in analysis than elsewhere, the client is asked to bring back a negative picture or memory, and have the incident come out some other way or alter the way in which it is perceived or held. Re-framing lends itself very well to a change of mental attitude. Alternatively the client may be encouraged to discover or find, some more overriding funny side to the memory of an experience. A useful way to do this is to ask the client to imagine he is with someone he greatly respects or admires.

When he has someone in mind - it could be someone he has never actually met but knows of - he is to imagine himself relating his experience to that person and as he does so the other person is taking him very seriously and then imagine that person begins to show amusement. The client should imagine the person smiling openly. Next, as the client continues to relate the matter to him he sees the person begin to laugh more and more until he loses his balance and falls to the ground, laughing hysterically whereupon the client too is to see it as equally funny and also to imagine falling to the ground laughing uncontrollably. Since this, like all these techniques is conducted in hypnosis, the funny aspect will override the former reaction to the original event and in thinking of that event subsequently it will be seen as far less important or even as a highly amusing event.

Another alternative to attitude change is for the client to imagine himself returning to a negative event and taking a leading role in it - particularly if he had been much younger at the time of the experience. He may see himself reassuring, cuddling, picking up, playfully punching his own younger self's arm; running his fingers through his hair in a comforting way; telling him it's okay; that he will grow up and be all right; it's just that others didn't understand or he didn't mean to do what he did and is wiser now. He may tell his former self that things are different; he is bigger now; more experienced and what happened then would never happen now and similar such suggestions may be used. He may hear himself using words to others that his former self would have liked to said.

As a further alternative, the client may be asked to imagine the same scene but be asked to imagine it was not himself, but some other person taking part and see the experience through from that perspective. Again, the client may bring into mind some other occasion where he had had a significant triumph and use the picture of that occasion to override the importance of the memory of the negative experience - rather like the 'laughing' method mentioned earlier, confidence and ego boosting reduce the effect of the original experience.

The client might also revalue others concerned in his pictured experience and consider what they were really like. He could imagine what they did wrong in their days, looking back at them now were they really intelligent, caring or understanding?. Were they happy? Were they really good judges of him? Were they right in what they did, or said? The reason for this last approach is that without realising it the original event had been taken at face value at the time, and no subsequent thoughts had updated or revalued the true situation. So too, the client might be invited to forgive them in the interest of freeing himself from them by doing so.

Future Pacing

In this the client is asked to imagine himself reacting or feeling in some much better way to a situation in which he has previously performed badly or felt uncomfortable with in the past. He is to see himself reacting and feeling in some wholly pleasing and satisfying way to a similar event in the future. For instance, the client who reports that he can drive well enough but has failed his driving test, say three times and feels he will never pass the test now. What the client is to do in hypnosis, is to see himself performing each individual driving skill well. He is to see this and feel his pleasure and confidence as he does do, and as if it were actually happening. The client concentrates in particular, on the areas of his driving where he otherwise feels less confident and particularly in areas where he failed in his previous driving test. For example, he should see himself arriving at just the right position to enter a roundabout, going through the gear changing and signalling procedures perfectly, see himself joining it, smoothly, confidently, feeling good, and turning off the roundabout smoothly and comfortably.

These mental exercises continue and culminate with his visualising and feeling immensely satisfied by being told by the examiner that he has passed the test. He then goes on to see himself with all the feelings he will have breaking the good news to others. He should have similar pictures of himself driving on his own feeling exhilarated with his new found freedom, especially if this is done just before a test it can have amazing effects particularly if failure in the past had been brought about by nervousness.

In this driving test illustration, a reinforcement may also be added by adjusting the client's attitude for he may, subconsciously, see such a test not just as of his driving skill but of himself as a whole or feel that the test is as much aimed at keeping him off the road as to any other reason. In short, as some personal challenge where the odds are stacked against him and reminding him of other failed challenges in his past. To overcome this negative attitude it is helpful in hypnosis to point out the test is really other things. It is an opportunity for him to be reassured and to have it confirmed to him that he is safe enough for his own good and before he finds himself left to his own devices some expert, who would rather pass him than fail him is confirming he really has a sufficient knowledge of driving to be safe particularly as he might well have as his passengers, valued loved ones he would wish to keep safe. Again, it can be put to him the awful hazards there would be if no such driving check-up were to exist and how dangerous it would then be with the roads full of untrained novice drivers learning by themselves as they drove, rather than a test of him, it is an opportunity to demonstrate his skills with all the pride of having mastered the art.

A session, built along the preceding lines and assuming the basic driving knowledge and skills do already exist, can have amazing results like the lady who had such a session two days before her ninth driving test. When she subsequently rang in with her good news she reported that everything had gone very smoothly. She had felt confident and calm and when the examiner had said he was passing her had told him that she knew he would, lent over, and gave him a kiss. (Leaning over and kissing the examiner is not to be recommended!)

Future pacing can be used, using the same principles, for such forthcoming events as interviews, meetings, important social occasions, public speaking, sporting events, anticipated stressful situations and to alter a person's reactions in many other ways. The driving test example, is just one illustration of this highly effective technique which, in itself, is really a re-programming exercise of course.

What Did The Guest Say?

Another good example of future pacing is illustrated in the case which follows. Attending her seventh session, the lady reported she was to entertain several friends to dinner that evening. She went on to explain she did this about every six months and that it was always a great strain on her. The staff she hired to help her were often either incompetent or seemingly uncooperative. The delivery of goods ordered to produce the meal, often being incomplete of poor quality or just late in arriving. It seemed to her that her friends who undertook similar entertaining in turn had no such difficulties.

In hypnosis she was invited to picture a series of events and do so as if they were actually happening. She was to visualise that her order had arrived fully and was in perfect condition; that the staff arrived and were cheerful, confident and talented. She was, in sequence to visualise seeing the meal's preparation going well with herself feeling happy and confident; in turn, to see guests arriving in good spirits and a perfect meal being served and appreciatively received. She was then to symbolise the accolade of success for the evening.

The lady reported that an important guest had said something but declined to tell me what was said. Returning for her eighth session, she stopped me halfway up the stairs to my office and most enthusiastically, reported that the entire occasion of the dinner had been an outstanding success in every way. However, she said: "It was almost eerie. I was amazed to hear that male guest suddenly say to me, exactly word for word what I had imagined him to say when I was last here". "Really", I said, "what did he say?" "I'm sorry", she said, "I couldn't repeat it!"

Of course, the Blow Away technique could have been used instead or even in addition to the future pacing technique, but prior to it. As always, it is a matter for personal judgement for no fixed rules can be applied.

Vocalisation

This is a further useful technique which can be used where, during analysis, the client comes across a memory of some experience in which something was not said, i.e., there was something the client should have, or desperately wanted to say at that time. In hypnosis he is directed to say or even shout those words out. An exercise frequently to result in tears with the release of the trapped emotion this brings. As an alternative, or in addition to saying or shouting unspoken words the client may be encouraged to hit out or bang his hands on something. For this we keep a 'hitting cushion', which is held in a comfortable position for him to strike. Great relief can be felt by the client in striking out in this way.

I've Got No Bust

A case example. A client reported her bust had never developed, and that she had a chest "As flat as that of a boy". In hypnosis she was taken back to the time that something was happening which caused her subconscious to prevent her breasts from developing. Following the 'one, two, three, click procedure, she immediately began seething with rage. She reported herself, aged ten, standing on a beach wearing only her knickers. Looking at her chest and smirking, was an eight year old boy. "What do you want to do?" she was asked, "hit him", she snapped back angrily "Then do it", she was commanded. (Thinking she would visualise her revenge) whereupon, much to her subsequent horror and embarrassment, she hit me instead knocking me flying. Hence the subsequent entrance of the hitting cushion. No serious harm was done, a lesson learnt and to the delight of the lady her bust began to develop.

Rebuilding

Rather like a tonic might be taken, to help speed recovery following some illness, a psychological tonic can similarly help mental recovery especially with a client who has endured long-term suffering, which had led in turn to a poor self-opinion, stress or self-guilt or, also with a client who is psychologically generally run down.

Analysis has released the inner causes of his condition but now he needs building up rather like one repairs a punctured tyre, but then has to re-inflate it, mending the puncture is the cure re-inflating it is the restitution. So too with the client, something may have to be put back, to give them a boost to their new start in life. I have a script I often use for this purpose. It may need some variation to fit a client more closely, but it can normally be used as it is and with a wide variety of clients. The script should be read with enthusiasm and emphasis - and of course with the client in hypnosis.

The Building Script

"(*client's name*) I want you to think of me as a friend, one who is helping you to become calmer and calmer, more and more relaxed, more and more at peace and you find that you do become calm, relaxed and peaceful; that a calm, relaxed, peaceful and self-confident feeling is beginning to grow and develop inside you; that your mind and body begin to run in total harmony together. It will surprise you and even amaze you to find how really peaceful and self confident you are. It will please you and delight you, as to how very calm, relaxed, peaceful and self-confident you actually have become".

"(*client's name*) A warm inner silence, a feeling of great inner calmness, relaxation, peacefulness and self-confidence is beginning to grow and develop inside you, moving gradually throughout the whole of your mind and body; flowing into every muscle, every limb, every part of you, and all the while I'm saying this (*client's name*), it doesn't matter if your mind should wander, if you should doubt what I say or even totally disbelieve it because you know, that to feel calm, relaxed, peaceful self-confident, and self-assured, are all feelings that you want to have. Since your subconscious is a great, loyal and immensely powerful inner friend, and there to work with you, you'll find that you do become calm, relaxed, peaceful, confident and self-assured - all with remarkably simple ease. (*client's name*) You take a great deal of pride and a great deal of pleasure, in the remarkably simple ease with which you actually do quit feeling tense and cease doubting yourself. You find it surprises you; it even amazes you that those feelings of inner peace, tranquillity and confidence that come from calmness, relaxation and self-assuredness, persist and last - persist and last - until they just become the normal way you are. (*client's name*) You find those feelings of inner calmness, relaxation, self-confidence and self-assurance actually become habits, welcome habits that open a whole new field of wonderful feelings, amazing successes and accomplishments. (*client's name*). You find that at first you can't even believe that it's you, feeling, acting and behaving in such a growing calm, relaxed, self-confident and self-assured way. All feelings and actions that delight and amaze you. You find that you become far more relaxed and confident than you ever thought possible!"

"How? Why? the answers are very simple indeed. You see, (*client's name*) for years you've been feeding your subconscious with negative self-doubts, self-denigration, anxiety, stress and self-criticism and since your subconscious mind is a loyal and dedicated part of you a part that follows your wishes and believes you; you became the way you thought. It's been a vicious circle; you doubted yourself and felt anxious; feelings which in turn became over time, accepted and believed to be true by your subconscious which in turn, negatively enhanced your feelings of anxiety and self-doubts in your conscious mind. Which, in turn, had been compounded there and fed back to your subconscious which in turn, were once again fed back to your conscious mind but, as even more powerfully reinforced misunderstandings so that any trivial set back or further misunderstanding, would once again feed your subconscious even more powerfully than before. (*client's name*) Consequently, you've been trying to fight your own mind in the past when you've tried to enforce and demand calmness, relaxation, confidence and self-assurance from within yourself because the negative programme, laid down by yourself, over the years had become too powerful, having fully accepted every set back, reinforcing your negative views of yourself and the world around you. (Then softly, slowly and sympathetically spoken) In all of this, (*client's name*) you are not to be blamed, condemned, found wanting, or criticised, because, above all else, you are a human being and we humans, not being machines can err, make mistakes, misunderstand things and sad to say too, at times even lose our way. (Now with enthusiastic emphasis) But! (*client's name*) in hypnosis, and even if you can't feel its presence, you find that you can reprogramme your subconscious, and not over years, but instantly because hypnosis enables us to go to the very heart of the matter, the nub of the issue, by allowing direct access to the keyboard of the subconscious computer - to erase one programme and to write in another and that's why it is so simple to make such welcome and wonderful changes. (Now motivationally spoken) It's not in the least bit difficult or complicated at all".

"Then, (continue with enthusiasm) (*client's name*) with a new self-confidence, new self-assurance and with a new inner sense of calmness, relaxation and peacefulness, comes surprising success, new and unbelievable self-achievements, a growing sense of determination and with each and every successful experience now compounding the wonderful new programme in the subconscious. And, because this is a programme you want and

183

enjoy, there's no conflict because you're no longer fighting your subconscious mind, but indeed instead, urging it on to even greater efforts which in turn, reinforces those same good qualities. Indeed (*client's name*) the wheel, so to speak, now turns in the opposite direction but runs freer, faster, smoother and far more productively than you can ever imagine possible! (*client's name*) It is for these simple, non-magical but logical reasons, that you find that you change and dramatically, (continue more softly) that you have wonderful feelings of calmness, relaxation and peacefulness. Feelings of self-confidence, self-assurance and determination. Feelings of an inner peace and tranquillity; an ability to cope, to be able to live with yourself as a goodly human being; to have a greater love and respect for yourself; a greater love and respect for yourself, that grows and grows and persists and lasts".

"You find that you take an immense pride and pleasure in your ability to be, and remain, calm and relaxed and to be more and more self-confident too (*client's name*) that a whole new field of wonderful experiences of calmness, relaxation, self-confidence and self-assurance has opened up to you. Experiences which last and persist, delight and amaze you. (*client's name*) you are now, nothing less than your true self, a self that grows stronger and stronger; a self you denied yourself until now, a self you welcome and admire. (*client's name*) So congratulations".

Role Reversal

This is another useful technique. In this, the client is to see himself as the therapist. In this role he is encouraged to tell his imagined client what he should do or how he is to act. The actual therapist is to extrapolate and emphasise the positive suggestions and advice that the client, in the role of therapist, gives to his imagined client.

The actual therapist is to watch for negative advice such as "That some person should be met and punched on the nose" and instead, guide him to give constructive advice. This constructive advice should be built up to a logical and enthusiastic pitch. Eventually the actual therapist, choosing his moment, is to state, in an emphatic voice. "So why don't you take the advice you've just given, yourself?" Conducted well, the client has no logical way out but to accept his own advice.

The Colour Technique

Colours can be taken to mean "I want" or "I have". Colour always has and continues, to play an important role in our lives. Since some animals are thought to be unable to detect colours it might even be considered that our ability to determine colours is another sense, in addition to the basic five. Colour is also widely used in the natural world of plants and insects. The flower produces colour to attract bees. Animals use colour for camouflage or to attract a mate. Insects, such as the wasp, use colour to protect themselves by pre-warning of danger. Colour effects human moods - indeed some people are highly reactive to it becoming excited, depressed or happier by some colours or combinations.

As a professional hypnotherapist I have developed a personal interpretation of colours and their meaning. Time and time again the theory is justified by experience because an insight into the theory and its foundation, consider our ancestors, so dependent on nature and interpreting colours to survive. Their dawn would be heralded by the sky lightening, becoming paler, turning to a virgin white or yellowish hue, 'another day', 'a new beginning'! The sky becomes blue, producing a sense of well-being. 'I feel good'. Soon it is time to hunt and gather, with the dangers of leaving the safety of the cave and settlement. Red for 'danger', 'determination' and 'challenge'!

Returning through the forest, the green of the grass that is the clearing of the forest at home, is eagerly looked out for and anticipated. Green for 'achievement', 'wanting' and 'needing'. The sky is to darken as the day closes. Dark Blue is the 'peace' of the sleep to come, with the rest it brings. In the black of the night is the end of the day, and in it occurs the partial loss of visual sense. Black is the 'mysterious', 'magical' and 'pessimism' in the mind. Brown is the 'messiness'. Pink the combination of the virginity of white, and the red of challenge, meaning 'female'. Orange the combination of the Red and Yellow interpretations, such as the determination for 'change'. Purple of Red and Blue (often meaning the magical belief, or a sexual matter that causes concern, or represents the conflict between the Red and Blue interpretations).

During analysis, this concept of colour meanings, can be used to obtain information from the subconscious, that can be most revealing and helpful. For instance, the therapist may say to his client. "I want your subconscious to pass me some important information, and that information will come in the answer to this question". (*client's name*) "I want you to imagine that you are standing on a carpet, look down now, and tell me what colour or colours is it made up of?" Alternatively the therapist might say to the client: "I want your subconscious to pass me an important message, your subconscious does that right now by putting a colour or colours into your mind". (*client's name*) "Tell me what you see". The colour or colours represent his subconscious feelings and thoughts, and are interpreted along the lines previously set out. For instance, 'Pink' - 'I'm female and proud of it' or more likely, 'I'm thinking of my mother' - but why?

Index

Chapter 1
Reincarnation and the Human Spirit

Chapter 2
The Oedipus and Electra Complexes

Chapter 3
Dealing Directly with the Subconscious

Chapter 4
The Induction of Hypnosis

Chapter 5
Conducting the Analysis

Chapter 6
Treating Children and Further Techniques

Useful Addresses

Training Courses and Seminars

These can be available to readers and are particularly recommended for students, councillors, members of the medical profession and practicing hypnotherapists. Subject to suitable volunteers attending, demonstrations of instant healing are attempted. Additionally, the concepts of the healing methods described in this series are discussed, developed and practiced. Training courses and seminars are offered subject to the availability of vacancies. Further information is readily available by sending a large stamped addressed envelope to:

John Howard,
Training Course Details,
P.O. Box 114,
Northampton NN2 6YW.

Psychotetic Lamps and Monitoring Meters

For details of this equipment, please send a large stamped addressed envelope to:

John Howard,
Dept. P and M,
P.O. Box 114,
Northampton NN2 6YW.

Registered Practitioners of Holistic Hypnotherapy

From February 1995 a list of qualified and experienced hypnotherapists who offer the therapies described in this series of books will be available free of charge. All enquiries <u>must</u> be accompanied by a large, stamped self-addressed envelope to:

John Howard (Practitioners' List),
P.O. Box 114,
Northampton NN2 6YW

Train yourself in Holistic Hypnotherapy

If you are encountering difficulties finding the other books which make up this present series, further information can be obtained direct from the publishers:

Brooklyn Publishing Group,
Moulton Park Business Centre,
Redhouse Road, Northampton NN3 1AQ.

Author's Appeal

As part of this series the author plans to publish an authorative book on the sexuality of the British public. The author would, therefore, be grateful to receive written contributions from readers, particularly on sexual practices, experiences and fantasies, fetishes, inclinations and features found sexually attractive in others. Contributions should be submitted, but please enclose your full name and address to (he will, of course, honour your anonymity in the book should you so wish but the subscriber must write to confirm - before any contributions are published - that he/she has the sole copyrights of such material):

John Howard (Author's Appeal),
P.O. Box 114, Northampton NN2 6YW.